The No-Drug Approach to Lowering Your Blood Pressure

by George E. Berkley, Ph.D.

Larchmont Books
New York

First printing: July, 1981

THE NO-DRUG APPROACH TO LOWERING YOUR BLOOD PRESSURE

Copyright © Larchmont Books, 1981

ISBN 0-915962-32-2

Printed in the United States of America

LARCHMONT BOOKS
*6 East 43rd Street
New York, N.Y. 10017
Tel., 212-949-0800*

Contents

*To Barbara and Hal Crosbie
in memory of many
happy moments spent
down on the Farm*

Author to Reader

Since blood pressure is a wide-ranging subject, encompassing a large and diverse number of medical issues, I have sought to simplify the presentation by using the question-and-answer approach. The "R" in the text is supposed to stand for you, the Reader. The "A" stands for me, the Author. Hopefully, you will find R posing the questions that you might ask. Hopefully, you will find A's answers reasonably clear and satisfactory. But if you don't find either of these to be the case, then I hope you won't get too upset. After all, anger would only raise your blood pressure, thus defeating not only your purpose, but also mine as well.

CHAPTER 1

Low Blood Pressure— The Key To Longer Life

R. Why do you call low blood pressure the key to longer life?

A. Because insurance company statistics clearly indicate that it is. Their figures show that people with lower blood pressures generally live longer than those whose blood pressures are higher.

R. I have heard that people who have high blood pressure tend to die earlier than others. Are you saying that even among people whose blood pressure is considered normal, the ones with the lower reading enjoy longer life expectancies?

A. That is exactly what I am saying. Take the case of a 35-year-old man whose blood pressure measures 130/90. He is considered to have quite normal blood pressure. However, he will, on the average, die four years sooner than a similarly aged male whose blood pressure is 120/80. If his blood pressure or BP, as we shall call it, rises to 140/95, it will still fall within the normal range by some standards. Yet he now can expect to die nine years earlier than his 120/80 counterpart.

R. You mean that if my blood pressure is lower than yours, I can be sure of living longer than you?

A. Not quite. Statistics don't work that way. They deal with groups, not individuals, and with probabilities rather than certainties. In any particular case, it may and often does happen that an individual lives longer than another individual whose BP is lower. However, the chances are that the reverse will occur. When it comes to longevity and, for that matter, health in general, the odds almost consistently favor those with lower blood pressure.

R. You seem to have used 120/80 as something of an ideal. But what about someone with a BP of 110/ 70? Does he or she have an advantage over someone with a reading of 120/80?

A. Yes. According to Dr. Edward D. Freis, a hypertension, or high blood pressure, specialist at the Veterans Administration Hospital in Washington, D.C., a reading of 120/80 is good but a reading of 110/70 is still better.

R. But can't a person's blood pressure get too low?

A. It can, but this happens only rarely. And it has to go down pretty far before it starts to become a problem. I know a woman physician whose blood pressure measures 90/48. Yet she feels, and claims to be, just fine. Of course, this might not make a desirable reading for everyone but it does indicate that BP can sink pretty low before we need to get concerned. It is blood pressure that is too high that is the real problem in modern life.

R. Just how many people suffer from blood pressure that is too high?

A. It depends on what we call high. For example, if we take 110/70 as the desirable figure, then a large majority of all the adults in this country have high blood pressure. Certainly, nearly all these people would, for the most part, benefit from reducing their blood pressure. If we take 120/80 as the cut-off figure—and Dr. Freis describes any reading greater than this as "not good"—then we would still include almost half of all adults. However, high blood pressure (HBP) or hypertension as it is called, is usually ascribed to higher levels. The National Health Survey of 1962 defined hypertension as anything over 160/95. It found that the BP of almost one out of five adult Americans exceeded at least one of these two figures. This finding prompted the survey to call hypertension the most common ailment in America today.

R. I imagine that when someone reaches this level his or her expected life span really becomes reduced.

A. You imagine correctly. A 35-year-old man with a BP of 160/100 will generally be classified as having only mild or moderate hypertension. Yet he can expect to die 16½ years earlier than can a male of the same age whose blood pressure is 120/80.

R. Hypertension usually takes its toll through caus-ing heart attacks and other heart-related problems, doesn't it?

A. Right again. Heart attacks kill one person every minute in the United States, and a man whose systolic or top blood pressure reading is 150 has more than twice the chance of becoming one of these victims than a man whose systolic pressure registers 120. With strokes, the difference, and the danger, become still more pro-nounced. Here the same 30-point difference in the sys-tolic reading makes the risk almost four times as great.

But high blood pressure, or HBP, can strike in other ways as well.

R. What are these other ways?

A. Hypertension will eventually cause kidney trou-ble in half of the people it afflicts. It will interfere with the kidney's filtering function, leading at first to fre-quent nightly trips to the bathroom. Later on, more severe problems can develop.

The brain is another organ which can suffer severe effects from high blood pressure. One or more of its tiny, fragile blood vessels can rupture, resulting in hem-orrhage and possible paralysis. Similar events can occur with the eyes, causing impaired vision.

Finally, high blood pressure may make an individual more vulnerable to cancer.

R. Cancer? I've never heard of that being caused by HBP. Are you sure about such a relationship?

A. We can not be absolutely sure that one causes the other but we have good evidence that a relationship exists. A research team at Northwestern University spent 14 years, from 1958 to 1972, tracking and analyzing the medical histories of nearly 1,500 men. They found that those with high blood pressure experienced a death rate from cancer that was *three times higher* than that suffered by those with normal blood pressure.

R. But couldn't that be due to the fact that those who had HBP were older or smoked cigarettes or were in some other way more likely to contract cancer? In other words, maybe the HBP people fell into the high cancer risk group for reasons that were unrelated to their blood pressure.

A. The study was a well-controlled one and these factors were taken into account. Yet, after due allowance for such things as age and cigarette smoking had been made, the startling discrepancy between the fatal cancer rates of those with HBP and those with normal BP still showed up. The team's leader, Dr. Alan R. Dyer, concluded that high blood pressure readings "are strongly related to subsequent mortality due to cancer."

R. All these facts and figures certainly make the case for lowering blood pressure clear and convincing. But before going on, I would like to know more about just what blood pressure is and what it does.

A. As you probably know, our bodies consist of billions of cells that require continual nourishment.

10

They obtain this nourishment from the blood which reaches them through a complex and convoluted circulatory system made up of arteries, veins, arterioles and capillaries.

R. I know that the arteries carry the blood from the heart and the veins transport it back to the heart, but I'm a bit hazy about the other two things you mention, the arterioles and the capillaries.

A. The capillaries are small, often quite tiny, blood vessels that receive the blood from the arteries and distribute it to the cells. The human body has millions of them.

R. What about the arterioles? I've never even heard of them before.

A. In some respects they play the crucial role. They are the smaller, outlying branches of the arteries that control the flow of blood to the capillaries.

R. And the heart functions as an engine keeping the whole system operating, right?

A. Right. Basically, it is a double pump. One part of it sends the old blood to the lungs for fresh oxygen; the other part takes this refreshed blood and sends it back through the circulatory system. Every day the heart must pump nearly 1,500 gallons of blood through well over 60,000 miles of blood vessels.

R. It sounds like an enormous job!

A. It is, yet the human body is so well designed that

our hearts under proper circumstances can fully and faithfully perform this task for more than a century without wearing out.

R. I gather, however, that if the heart doesn't exert itself enough, that too could prove dangerous.

A. Absolutely. The absence of all blood pressure is death. However, the overwhelming majority of us could function well even if our hearts exerted considerably less pressure than they already do. The figures indicate that over 90% of all Americans could lower their systolic blood pressure by more than 10 points and only benefit as a result. Until the systolic or top figure dips below 90, blood pressure that is too low does not usually become a cause for concern.

R. What causes blood pressure to become too high?

A. To begin with, medicine makes a distinction between what it calls essential and what it calls secondary hypertension. Secondary hypertension results from various deficiencies and defects elsewhere in the body such as in the kidneys, adrenal glands, the nervous system, etc. Frequently these conditions can be remedied or at least mitigated. When this happens, the hypertension will often disappear.

R. What about essential hypertension?

A. This is the real problem. First, because it covers 85% of all hypertension—only 15% can be classified as secondary—and secondly, because its cause and cure remains much more illusive. We do know that hardening of the arteries (arteriosclerosis) can create or at least 'aggravate hypertension. When the arteries lose their elasticity, they do not "give" as much and this forces the heart to pump harder in order to discharge its mission. Fatty deposits on the walls of the arteries will have the same effect for now the heart must exert itself to squeeze the blood through narrower and tighter blood vessels. This condition is called atherosclerosis and should not be confused with arteriosclerosis or the hardening of the arteries cited above. However, both conditions tend to elevate blood pressure.

When any hardening or narrowing of the arteries forces the heart to work harder, the heart itself will eventually respond by enlarging. This enlargement may well prompt it to pump more blood than the blood vessels can accommodate, thus leading to increased danger from heart attacks, strokes and other serious complications.

To make the situation still more complicated, a reverse effect occurs. Increased blood pressure can damage the arteries and arterioles, causing them to become less elastic. This in turn will force the heart to pump yet harder, thus requiring an increased level of pressure.

R. But where does it all begin?

A. No one can say for sure. Modern medicine does not know all the factors that cause elevated blood pressure. Some of these factors are apparently genetic or inborn since some people actually seem programmed for high blood pressure.

However, an abundance of research has emerged, much of it relatively recently, which points out a lot of fairly simple steps that almost anyone can take with excellent expectations that at least some of them will bring lower blood pressure, and thus the benefits that such lower blood pressure apparently confers.

R. Well, I now feel I know more about blood pressure than I did before, but I still have a lot of questions I would like to ask before we go on to discuss the ways and means of lowering it. For one thing, why are two different numbers used to measure blood pressure?

A. The first or top number measures the systolic pressure or the pressure that the heart is exerting when it is actually pumping. The bottom number is called the diastolic, and it measures the heart's pressure between beats or when it is at rest. This means that the top or systolic pressure is the maximum pressure, while the diastolic or bottom number represents the minimum. This will explain why the bottom number is invariably smaller.

R. Is it true that the bottom number is the most important one?

A. There used to be some feeling that the diastolic reading was more critical than the systolic. However, today most doctors regard both as equally important. In any case both generally move together in the same direction. That is, an increase in one will generally be followed by an increase in the other and vice-versa.

R. You have quoted one expert as saying that anything over 120/80 is "not good." But doesn't our blood pressure tend to go up the longer we live? What about the popular saying that a person's blood pressure should equal 100 plus his age?

A. In most western countries peoples' blood pressure does tend to rise until the age of 55 or so. However, there are groups in the South Pacific, South America and Africa whose blood pressure remains the same throughout life. Even in this country, some five per cent of the population retains the same level of blood pressure in old age as they had in youth. The fact that blood pressure usually does go up with age does not mean it must or should go up. Dr. Josef P. Hrachovec, a research physician at the Gerontology Center at the University of Southern California says in his book, *Keeping Young and Living Longer*, that "low blood pressure throughout life is truly and perfectly normal." It's also most desirable and, in many cases, perfectly attainable.

R. What about children? Can they ever suffer from high blood pressure?

A. They can and they do. A few years ago a pediatrician at Children's Hospital in Los Angeles reported finding HBP in one per cent of all babies tested. This may not seem like a high figure, but as the pediatrician pointed out, it is higher than the incidence of many other childhood ailments. *The New York Times*, in commenting on the report, observed that "the unexpected discovery that infants are susceptible to adult forms of hypertension represents a new dimension of one of the nation's most serious health problems." (October 15, 1974).

R. Doesn't heredity play a large role in blood pressure?

A. It seems to. According to the American Medical Association, if one parent has hypertension, there is a

50 per cent chance that at least one of their offspring will eventually develop it. If both parents suffer from hypertension, then the chance that one or more of their children will become similarly afflicted rises to 90 per cent. Thus, heredity factors may create a predisposition toward high blood pressure. But, the fact that you may be more susceptible to it than someone else only means that you should take greater precautions to avert or control it. And don't forget that millions upon millions of Americans whose parents had normal blood pressure are nevertheless afflicted with this ailment today.

R. Can't a person's blood pressure rise momentarily but then fall back to a normal level? If I have my blood pressure taken and it registers a high figure, couldn't this be only a temporary condition?

A. It could. It usually takes more than one reading to accurately determine blood pressure. If your BP registers a high reading, then you should try to have it checked again, perhaps several times over the following weeks. Still, any high reading should alert you to the need or at least the desirability of taking precautionary measures.

R. What, then, are the symptoms of high blood pressure?

A. The most common is dizziness. Others are fatigue, heart palpitations, headaches and flushing in the face. These are the usual symptoms when they occur. The trouble is that they don't always occur. The victim frequently feels just fine. This is why HBP is sometimes called "the silent killer."

16

R. How about the person with blood pressure that is too low? How does he feel? Also, what causes overly low blood pressure?

A. People whose blood pressure has sunk too low often feel tired and sluggish. Like HBP sufferers, however, they may also experience dizzy spells. In their case, such spells are more likely to occur when they shift positions such as standing up after having been seated for a period of time.

Low blood pressure, in the sense of being too low, is rarely a chronic condition. It can be brought on by loss of blood, dehydration, malfunctioning of the adrenal glands or illness generally. Correct the condition and you will usually send the BP back to safe levels.

R. What makes women so fortunate in this respect?

A. Again, modern science lacks all the answers. We do know that at birth an infant boy's blood vessels will have a much thicker internal lining than a girl's. Remembering what we discussed earlier regarding BP and ths size of the circulatory passages may thus give us one clue to the disparity in their blood pressures. Another factor may lie in diet. Women seem to eat less of the foods that, as we shall see, elevate blood pressure and more of those foods which tend to bring it down. Furthermore, as we shall also see, the mineral magnesium plays a part in blood pressure management, and according to one researcher, Mildred Seelig, M.D., women seem to metabolize magnesium better than men.

But one thing is important to keep in mind. The difference in BP between men and women is most pronounced in the earlier years. After menopause, women's blood pressure readings tend to come closer to men's.

After age 60, the difference, while still there, is nowhere near as great as it once was.

The impact of this change reveals itself in the heart attack rate. Up to the age of 40, the heart attack rate for men in actually 24 times greater than it is for women. After age 40, the gap between the sexes shrinks substantially.

R. What causes this change in middle life?

A. Before menopause, women produce a lot of estrogen, a hormone which, so it is believed, helps to keep blood pressure low. After menopause the production of estrogen falls off sharply.

R. Can't women take estrogen injections?

A. They can and for a long time they did. But the popularity of such shots has fallen off in the face of numerous reports as to their adverse side effects. Such injections, so some research indicates, produce an appreciably greater risk of cancer, among other things.

R. So most women, too, have a stake in learning to lower their blood pressure?

A. Absolutely.

R. Are some races more vulnerable to high blood pressure than others?

A. Apparently. For example, one out of three American Blacks can expect to suffer from high blood pressure. This is about double the rate for American Whites.

R. Isn't this due to the greater stress which characterizes so much of Black life in this country?

A. This could be the case. Certainly, Blacks in Africa show no disposition in this direction. It could also come from the fact that Blacks lived for so many centuries in an environment that contrasts so sharply with that of the present-day United States. In doing so, they may have acquired certain physiological characteristics which make it more difficult for them to adapt to our present environment. For example, almost all doctors accept the fact that salt has an adverse effect on blood pressure and we know that salt was and is in short supply in many parts of Africa. This may have caused many Africans to become accustomed to less salt than Europeans and therefore to become less able to handle the tremendous amounts of salt in the current American diet.

On February 4, 1979, the *New York Times* reported the results of an interesting 10-year study conducted in Detroit. It revealed that the darker a Black person's skin, the more likely he or she was to have HBP. There was a direct relationship between pigmentation and blood pressure. As you probably know, over 90 per cent of all Blacks in this country have had one or more white ancestors. Thus, it may be that those Blacks with fewer or no white forebears are more vulnerable to HBP. In any case, those who conducted the study felt the greater emotional stress which Blacks are subjected to in our culture was only one factor in the situation and not the whole problem.

R. Did the same type of skin-color relationship hold true for Whites?

A. No. For Whites the reverse is true: the darker the skin color, the less likelihood of HBP.

R. Why?

A. No one knows. However, as already noted and as will be seen later on, some foods tend to lower blood pressure while others tend to raise it. The "good" foods in this respect more frequently crop up in the diets of those from Southern Europe; the "bad" foods are more prevalent in the diets of those from Northern Europe. Since Southern Europeans tend to be darker than Northern Europeans, this might possibly explain some or even all of the difference. But, again, no one can say for sure.

R. What's wrong with taking drugs for HBP? Aren't they effective?

A. In a technical sense they can be quite effective. There is no question that doctors have succeeded in lowering the BP of many people through using one or more of the 50 or so drugs currently available on the market for this purpose. But these drugs do not always work, and even when they do, they usually produce serious side effects.

R. What are some of these side effects?

A. Nausea, fatigue, sexual impotence in men, and a host of others. Most of these drugs also deplete the body's supply of potassium and, as will be explained later on, the supplements which doctors often prescribe to compensate for this don't always work too well. Some drugs even tend to wash vitamin B6 out of the system.

A much more severe side effect is cancer. Studies at Oxford University in England, the Boston University Medical School and at the University of Utah Medical School have all pointed to this danger. As a matter of fact, the Food and Drug Administration in September, 1974, warned physicians that women taking drugs containing reserpine, a commonly used substance in BP control, ran a risk of breast cancer that was two or three times greater than that of other women.

R. Does that mean that people with HBP should not take drugs?

A. By no means. But they should simultaneously seek to lower their blood pressure through more natural methods so that they can reduce their need for such medication. Some may reach the point where they will not need drugs at all. Certainly, many have already done so.

R. If these more natural methods are so effective as you claim, why don't doctors make greater use of them?

A. Doctors usually do tell their HBP patients to give up cigarettes, cut down on salt and, if they are overweight, to reduce. These are all useful admonitions although, as we shall learn, there is much more to be said about all of them. But, in general, most doctors show little interest in these other methods of blood pressure control even when, as is often the case, they are backed up by scrupulous scientific research. Indeed, most doctors don't even know about most of this research.

21

R. Why don't they?

A. To understand why they don't, you must first understand that doctors are trained and oriented to the more technical aspects of medicine. Drugs, surgery and the use of various technological devices constitute for them the more challenging parts of their profession. Don't forget, also, that doctors are usually too busy to read very much except brochures from the drug companies. And don't forget that these simpler approaches could actually endanger their livelihood, for people could use most of these on their own without even going to a doctor.

R. Could you be more specific?

A. Certainly. As you will see in the pages that follow, there is a lot one can do to lower blood pressure through nutrition alone. Yet most doctors, sad to say, are nutritional nincompoops. A study of doctors at the Harvard Medical School showed that, on average, they know just a tiny bit more about nutrition than the average secretary at the Harvard Medical School. This at least was true unless the secretary was overweight. The overweight secretaries, so it seems, actually knew a bit more about nutrition than did the doctors at this, the nation's most prestigious medical school.

In 1979, the weekly tabloid *National Enquirer* asked a professor of nutrition at Cornell University to devise a test which the paper then gave to 120 doctors attending a conference of the American Medical Association. The result? None of the doctors answered nine out of 10 questions correctly, and so none got A's. Two managed to get B's, two got C's, and eight others succeeded in getting D's. The remaining 90 percent flunked the test completely.

The questions they missed included naming the amount of iron needed by the average woman in her daily diet and picking the highest and lowest calorie items from a list of common foods. When given another list of 10 foods and asked to pick from it the six high-salt items, only two out of the 120, or less than 2 per cent, managed to do so.

As with nutrition, so with many other areas of health that can help high blood pressure. The average doctor simply doesn't know and, in all too many cases, doesn't care to know, what such procedures have to offer.

R. But surely not all doctors fall into this category?

A. There are several hundred physicians in the United States who are deeply involved in developing simpler and more natural remedies for various ailments, including high blood pressure. Fortunately, their numbers are growing. And, as we shall see, some of them are among the more eminent and esteemed members of their profession. As yet, however, they constitute far less than one per cent of all practicing physicians in this country.

R. What should I do if I can't find one of these physicians?

A. Stick with the one you have as long as he or she seems reasonably competent. In the meantime, start taking some responsibility for your own health and start taking advantage of some of the information available for doing so. Check everything with your doctor if you wish, but do not count on an enthusiastic endorsement. Since he will most likely not know about this data and will feel somewhat threatened by your presenting it to him—after all, you are, in effect, accusing him of not knowing everything he ought to know—he may deride and dismiss it. But unless he can give you medically sound reasons why you should not utilize it, then go ahead and do so. You may be, indeed you probably will be, pleasantly surprised by the results.

CHAPTER 2

It's Not Just Salt

R. Why do doctors usually recommend cutting down on salt as a way of lowering high blood pressure?

A. Because salt has been shown to correlate with HBP in both laboratory animals and man. Forgetting for a moment the laboratory animals and focusing on man, we find, for example, that in parts of northern Japan where over an ounce of salt is consumed by the average person every day, high blood pressure is common and about one-half of the population dies from strokes. But in parts of Africa where virtually no salt is consumed, there is virtually no high blood pressure and virtually no heart ailments as well.

R. What about this country?

A. The same relationship holds true. One study compared a group of people with HBP with another group whose blood pressure was normal. It was found that those in the hypertension or HBP group were eating, on the average, about four times as much salt as those in the normal BP group.

R. But don't some people use a good deal of salt without getting high blood pressure?

A. Yes, some people can tolerate much more salt than can the rest of us. Even whole groups may enjoy remarkable resistence to salt. For example, farmers in northern Thailand ingest somewhat more salt than we do but enjoy normal blood pressure into old age. Nevertheless, salt does tend to elevate blood pressure in most people.

R. What is it in salt that makes it so harmful?

A. Salt is actually a chemical compound called sodium chloride. It's the sodium that causes the trouble.

R. But I have heard that sodium is a mineral that is essential to human health.

A. You have heard correctly. But only a small amount is required, perhaps about 500 milligrams a day. Five hundred milligrams is only half a gram, and it takes 28 grams to make an ounce. So you see it takes less than one-fiftieth of an ounce to supply all the sodium that the human body needs. Amounts greatly in excess of this can prove damaging and even dangerous.

R. Just how does excess sodium cause or aggravate high blood pressure?

A. Modern medicine is not absolutely sure but the belief is that sodium works its nefarious way by causing the body to retain water. This retained fluid in turn causes the tissues of the arteries to swell, and this forces the heart to work harder to drive the blood through the now narrowed passageways. You will recall from the previous chapter that any tightening of the arterial passages will require more pressure to push the blood through them.

R. How many Americans consume excess salt or sodium?

A. Most of us, and this is probably one reason why most of us have higher blood pressures than we should have for maximum health.

R. Where does all this salt come from?

A. From everywhere. In our modern society there almost seems to be a conspiracy to put unneeded and undesirable quantities of salt into our food supply and hence into our bodies.

R. Could you be more specific?

A. Certainly. Let's start right from the beginning, that is, from birth. Most Americans alive today were raised on cow's milk, not mother's milk. As it so happens, cow's milk has four to five times as much sodium as human breast milk. Thus, the typical baby starts out by receiving much more salt than he or she needs.

Baby foods will customarily compound the problem, for these preparations usually harbor high levels of salt. As a matter of fact, one laboratory experiment found that young rats developed fatal high blood pressure after being exposed to the degree of dietary salt found in commercial baby foods. Adjusting for weight differences, the typical baby being fed such foods along with cow's milk is getting what for an adult would be the equivalent of 23 grams of sodium a day. *This is almost 50 times more than is required for health.* Indeed, it approaches the level of salt consumption found in those sections of northern Japan that I mentioned earlier.

R. What about the typical adult diet?

A. It too is saturated with salt. For example, 100 grams of fried bacon will contain 2,400 milligrams of sodium. In other words, less than four ounces of this popular breakfast food will supply almost five times as much sodium as we need for an entire day. Remember that there are 1,000 milligrams to a gram and about 28 grams to an ounce, and the human requirement is only 500 milligrams or half a gram a day.

R. What about other meats?

A. Most of them are not as bad as fried bacon in this respect, but many of them come close. The same 100 grams of corned beef gives us 1,300 milligrams of salt. From the same amounts of ham or frankfurters we get 1,100 milligrams, and from pork sausage 740.

R. Are there any meats which are low in sodium?

A. Chicken and turkey rank lowest, especially the latter and more especially the white meat. The white meat of turkey will supply only 40 milligrams of sodium per 100 grams, while the dark meat provides 92. For chicken the figures are 65 for the light and 90 for the dark. Lean pork will contain 55 milligrams, lean lamb 90 and lean veal 100.

R. What about fish? I imagine that it has much more salt than meat.

A. Not necessarily. Fresh fish filets are actually quite low in sodium. For example, four ounces of cod will only yield 60 milligrams, while the same amount of flounder will provide 70. Shellfish have higher sodium values. Four ounces of lobster, for instance, contain about 270 milligrams of sodium. However, even this amount is, as we have seen, lower than that of many meats. Furthermore, some shellfish are fairly low in sodium. Oysters have only about 140 milligrams for four ounces.

R. So most forms of fish are fairly safe?

A. By no means. Fish that has been smoked or canned or processed in any way is likely to have large amounts of salt. A four-ounce can of tuna will supply almost twice our daily requirement.

R. Does that mean we should avoid all canned fish?

A. I hate to say so, for some of them offer us economical and easy ways of obtaining what are otherwise very nutritious foods. Tuna is a good source for a certain trace mineral that, as we shall learn in the next chapter, is most useful in controlling blood pressure. Sardines, which are also packed with salt, are another healthful food. However, in consuming such foods, we should take care to wash them *thoroughly* in water before putting them on the table.

R. You mentioned that cow's milk is quite high in sodium. Does that mean that we should not drink milk?

A. What I said was that it contains much more sodium than breast milk. An eight-ounce glass of milk has a little over 100 milligrams of sodium. While milk can not be called a low-sodium food, it is not unduly high in sodium either. And it is quite nutritious, though not as much so as the Dairy Council would have us believe.

R. What about other dairy products?

A. With cheeses there is a good deal of difference depending on whether they are natural or processed. As you might suspect, the processed kinds contain much more salt, indeed, more than double as much as the natural ones. But even most natural cheeses tend to be somewhat salty. Four ounces of a typical one will contain 750 milligrams of salt.

As for butter, a four-ounce stick of the commonly used variety has 1,000 milligrams or one gram of sodium. We can reduce this amount by about 12 per cent through substituting what is called sweet butter, and we can reduce it by a full 99 per cent, to about 10 milligrams, by substituting unsalted butter.

R. What about margarine?

A. Margarine is worse. It has about 10 per cent more salt than regular butter.

R. What about other things such as fruits, vegetables and grains?

A. In general, all of these tend to be quite low in sodium unless they have been processed; then the damage can be great. Kidney beans, to take one example, are only moderate suppliers of salt. But four ounces of canned kidney beans contain over 600 milligrams of sodium. When it comes to bread products, we find that soda crackers provide as much sodium as ham or frankfurters. Most breakfast cereals also have a lot of salt.

R. Can I assume, then, that all unprocessed fruits, vegetables and flour will be low in sodium?

A. Not quite. A few of these items, fortunately very few, do have high amounts of it. Probably the most pernicious are green olives and pickles. A table at the back of the book will list the sodium content of most foods in common use.

R. Are there any other sources of salt in our food supply?

A. There are lots of them. They seem to pop up everywhere we turn. Many preservatives are heavily composed of sodium. Their names, such as sodium nitrate and sodium benzoate, reveal this. What's more, our water supply is becoming heavily salted.

R. How so?

A. One way is through the use of water softeners. These agents remove many valuable minerals from our water. At the same time they increase its sodium content. Softened water can have 10 times as much sodium as the water originally contained.

Another and increasingly worrisome problem is the

use of salt to counteract the effects of ice on roads in the winter time. Northern states now use nine million tons of salt each winter for this purpose.

R. How can this affect the water?

A. It seeps into the soil and from there into the water supply. Areas that use much more salt than others consistently show more salt in their water. And this is having its effect on the blood pressure of their inhabitants. Some University of Massachusetts scientists did a five-year comparison study of two Boston suburban towns, one with a high salt level in its drinking water, the other with a level that was much lower. They found that high school students in the high salt community averaged blood pressure readings similar to persons who were two to 10 years older. High salt concentrations also tend to destroy trees and other forms of vegetation.

It is somewhat ironic that up to about 300 years ago mankind frequently had to struggle to obtain sufficient sources of salt. Wars were even waged over rights to salt deposits. Today, those of us in the industrialized world at least live in salt-saturated societies and suffer from this overabundance.

R. But salt does add flavor to food. Wouldn't eating be a pretty dull process without it?

A. Not necessarily. The big problem is that we have become accustomed to consuming so much salt that we have begun to lose our taste for it. Therefore, we require more and more of it on our food. A study done in 1962 showed that high blood pressure patients cannot taste salt as well as those with normal blood pressure. The researchers felt, logically enough, that this could be a factor in prompting such people to ingest excessive amounts of it. After a person has become accustomed to a low-salt diet, he usually finds that many ordinary foods taste too salty.

I should also like to point out that there are many substitutes that we can use for salt.

R. Such as?

A. Well, first of all there are the condiments which are labeled "salt substitutes" and are sold in most health food stores as well as in some supermarkets. These often contain potassium chloride, and potassium choloride, as we will shortly see, can do double duty. That is, not only can it keep us from using salt but at the same time it adds something to our diet that will aid our blood pressure control mechanism.

Then there are all the various herbs and spices that are available. Unlike salt, these can actually promote health. For example, take chili powder. Some research suggests that the chili pepper can dilate the blood vessels, making them somewhat more resistant to hardening. Try some on your eggs next time, along with some paprika or nutmeg or curry powder or any combination of them all. For your tomatoes you may prefer basil and thyme. Experiment, and you will come up with a lot of acceptable alternatives to salt.

R. The case against salt seems pretty strong. However, the title of this chapter, "It's Not Just Salt", implies that something else may also be involved. What is it?

A. I thought you'd never ask. It appears that salt or rather sodium has a natural enemy that can neutralize much of its destructiveness. That enemy is potassium.

As far back as 1928 the *Canadian Medical Association Journal* carried a research report to this effect. The researchers claimed to have found that "potassium salt regularly produced a decline in blood pressure," while sodium salt just as regularly produced a rise in blood pressure.

Through the years additional research tended to bear out this sensational but little-noticed finding. In 1951 it was found that the blood pressure of laboratory animals could be raised not only by feeding them lots of salt but also by *not* feeding them any foods with potassium. In 1953, it was reported that volunteer human research subjects placed on potassium-deficient diets would tend to develop HBP. It was also learned that people eating as much salt as they wished would excrete in their urine nine times as much potassium as those whose salt consumption had been limited. This again pointed up the natural antagonism between the two minerals and suggested that one way sodium might elevate the blood pressure would be to drive out potassium.

R. Sounds intriguing but I'm not yet completely convinced.

A. Well, there's more. In 1969, Herbert Langford, M.D., a professor of medicine at the University of Mississippi Medical School, undertook, with some associates, to survey blood pressure levels among high school students. They failed to establish any distinct and significant relationship between the amount of sodium excreted in a student's urine and his or her blood pressure. But what they did establish was a marked relationship between the proportion of potassium to sodium and the subject's blood pressure. As Dr. Langford put it, "what we have found, and most clearly, was that the sodium/potassium ratio correlated with blood pressure." (*Prevention*, November, 1978.) In other words, the higher the amount of potassium *in proportion to the amount of sodium* which a student excreted, the lower his or her blood pressure was likely to be.

All these research reports were capped off by a fairly definitive study that was disclosed at a conference of the American Heart Association in the Spring of 1978. The researchers in this study had tested the potassium and sodium levels of almost 2,000 people, both Black and White, in three different American cities. Although some relationship between sodium levels and high blood pressure did emerge, the most significant relationship was, again, the potassium/sodium ratio. As one of the researchers put it, "the people studied who excrete more potassium in relation to sodium have lower blood pressure." Apparently it's as simple as that.

R. Does this mean we can eat all the salt we want as long as we eat lots of potassium along with it?

A. Not quite. What it does indicate is that lowering salt consumption may not be enough. What is needed is a two-pronged war, so to speak, in which we lower our salt consumption while we increase our potassium intake. On the other hand, sufficient amounts of potassium in our diets may enable some of us to be a bit more liberal in our salt intake than we might otherwise want to be.

R. You spoke earlier about how our normal Western diet was overly supplied with salt. Is this the case with potassium, too?

A. Far from it. As already noted, salt and potassium seem to be natural enemies. The more salt we have added to our foodstuffs, the more potassium we have driven out. For example, 3½ ounces of fresh, raw green peas provide 316 milligrams of potassium and only 2 milligrams of sodium. This is a most favorable ratio. But what happens after the peas are canned? They will then contain 236 milligrams of sodium and only 96 milligrams of potassium. There has been an almost total turnaround in their potassium/sodium ratio.

Take what happens to the whole wheat in Wheaties, one of the better commercial breakfast foods. A pound of whole wheat contains 1,700 milligrams of potassium and a mere 9 milligrams of sodium. A pound of Wheaties, on the other hand, has almost 4,700 milligrams of sodium and no potassium at all!

Finally, it should be noted that simply cooking vegetables or grains such as rice in water can destroy much of their potassium. The mineral leaches into the water during the cooking process.

R. *One would imagine from what you say that not only are we a salt-saturated society but also a potassium-deficient one.*

A. There is some evidence that this is indeed the case. The magazine *Geriatric Focus* published in 1969 the results of a careful survey of senior citizens in a community near Glasgow, Scotland. The study found that more than half of these people were not getting the amounts of potassium necessary to meet *minimum* standards.

R. *What about the situation in this country?*

A. It is most probably worse. Fast foods and processed foods generally are more heavily consumed here than in Scotland. These foods, as we have seen, tend to have the worst potassium-to-sodium ratios.

R. What about the fact that the people in the Scottish survey were elderly? Would the situation regarding younger adults today be better?

A. More likely it, too, would be worse. Younger adults are more used to processed and, especially, fast foods and probably consume more of them. Also, younger people are more physically active and physical activity, as we shall learn when we examine exercise, increases the body's need for potassium. Finally, don't forget that this survey was taken in the late 1960s. It is now the 1980s and the potassium-to-sodium ratio in the average diet in nearly all Western countries has undoubtedly worsened.

R. Doctors often give their high blood pressure patients potassium supplements. Is it because of the facts you have just recounted?

A. Not really. Doctors frequently prescribe diuretics to people with HBP. These diuretics tend to flush out salt but also potassium as well. The potassium supplements are designed to prevent a serious potassium deficiency which can lead to muscle weakness and other problems. They are not given with the intention of trying to build a maximum potassium-to-sodium ratio. Furthermore, as we shall see in the next chapter, these diuretics may also cause the body to lose another valuable mineral in addition to potassium and no supplementation is usually given to make up for this possible loss.

R. Are you suggesting, then, that HBP patients should not take the potassium supplements their doctors prescribe for them?

A. Certainly not. It is never my intention to recommend to any person not to follow his or her doctor's advice. What I am suggesting is that the vast majority of Americans, whether they are on medication for HBP or enjoy what is called normal blood pressure, could benefit by eating more high-potassium, low-sodium foods.

R. What are these foods?

A. To begin with, fruits. Nearly all of them have a high potassium-to-sodium ratio. Three of the best are bananas, grapes or raisins, and oranges. Concerning this last fruit item, it is interesting to observe that when the first group of astronauts were sent into space, they were given a commercial orange-like preparation containing synthetic vitamin C to drink, instead of real orange juice. When they came back, they were found to be potassium deficient. Prunes are another good source of potassium as are watermelon, apples, dates, apricots or just about anything in the fruit department.

Many vegetables, indeed most of them, also provide desirable potassium-to-sodium ratios. Potatoes, particularly when baked and eaten with some of the skin, give ample amounts of potassium with almost no sodium. Rice does the same. An American physician, Dr. Walter Kempner, once achieved great success in reducing HBP by putting his patients on a rice and fruit diet.

Unsalted nuts and seeds are also good. So is molasses. And bran may be best of all. In the appendix you will find the list I referred to earlier which provides the sodium content of various common foods.

Salt and sodium conversions

Grams to milligrams	**Multiple weight in grams by 1,000**
Sodium into salt (NaCl) equivalent	**Milligrams of sodium content ÷ 0.40 = milligrams of salt**
Salt into sodium	**Milligrams of salt × 0.40 = milligrams of sodium**
Sodium in milligrams to sodium in milliequivalents[1]	**Milligrams of sodium ÷ 23 (atomic weight of sodium) = milliequivalents of sodium**
Milliequivalents of sodium to milligrams of sodium	**Milliequivalents of sodium × 23 = milligrams of sodium**

[1]Medical prescriptions are often given as milliequivalents (mEq).
Source: "The Sodium Content of Your Food," Home and Garden Bulletin No. 233, USDA, August, 1980.

CHAPTER 3

Other Minerals
That Help - and Hurt

R. What are these other minerals which affect blood pressure?

A. Let's begin with the one most people are most familiar with, calcium.

R. Calcium? I thought that was primarily needed by babies and growing children for their bones and teeth?

A. Actually, people of all ages need calcium for this purpose and, as a matter of fact, older adults may need it more than younger ones. The U.S. Public Health Service recommends an abundant supply of calcium for anyone over 40 to promote bone strength. The frequency with which older people fracture their bones attests to their need for increased calcium. Women, by the way, tend to suffer more from this problem than do men.

R. Okay. But that still doesn't say what calcium does to affect blood pressure.

A. Actually, calcium does not *directly* affect blood pressure. However, it does play a part in some of the things that may cause or aggravate HBP. It also can help alleviate some of the consequences of HBP.

R. How so?

A. We know that stress and its many manifestations can raise blood pressure. Calcium helps reduce stress. According to Dr. W. M. Ringsdorf, Jr., a Professor of Medicine at the University of Alabama Medical School, calcium does this so well that it can even replace certain drugs such as tranquilizers and sleeping pills. He believes that at least one out of every four Americans suffer from a calcium deficiency, and that this has produced a good deal of the nervousness, irritability and insomnia which characterize so much of modern life.

R. Is Dr. Ringsdorf the only medical practitioner who makes such a claim?

A. No, numerous others who have looked into the subject say the same. A California physician, Dr. Richard Huemer, believes that calcium deficiencies may be even more widespread and that they are responsible for a host of stress symptoms. It seems that our nervous systems as well as our bones and teeth require calcium and all too often they fail to obtain enough of it.

R. What about calcium's role in mitigating the consequences of high blood pressure?

A. As discussed earlier, high blood pressure, or even simply higher blood pressure, makes an individual more liable to heart ailments. Calcium appears to prevent or at least reduce the seriousness of such ailments. A study at the University of Birmingham in England has brought this out. The researchers sought to relate the dietary intake of certain nutrients with death from various natural causes. They found that the strongest single relationship was the one which existed between calcium in the diet and heart disease. And the relationship was a negative one which means that the less calcium in the diet, the more likelihood there was of dying from heart trouble. There are several other studies which suggest the same thing.

R. Just how does calcium protect the heart?

A. In more ways than one, most likely. Calcium is important for the normal contraction and relaxation of muscles, and the heart, though it functions as a pump, is actually a muscle. So this is one way in which calcium could help the heart. Another way is through lowering cholesterol and other fats in the blood.

R. I have heard that a high level of cholesterol in the blood can make one more susceptible to heart trouble but I've never heard that calcium could reduce it.

A. There have been several studies which have shown this to be the case. Many of them were carried out in England but one notable one was undertaken at St. Vincent's Hospital in Montclair, New Jersey in the late 1960s. There, 10 men and women suffering from high cholesterol levels were given large amounts of calcium daily. At the end of a year, their average cholesterol level had fallen by nearly 25 per cent.

R. Any side effects?

A. None whatever. Indeed, other studies indicate that calcium does not even lower cholesterol in people whose cholesterol level is already normal. One might say that it tends to normalize cholesterol.

R. How much calcium do we need to obtain these benefits?

A. The Food and Nutrition Board recommends 800 milligrams for adults and young children and larger quantities for youngsters 11 years of age and up. The 10 people involved in the New Jersey experiment received 2,000 milligrams a day. Dr. Ringsdorf recommends a daily adult intake of 1,200 milligrams a day.

R. Milk and other dairy products are our prime source of calcium, are they not?

A. They may be our prime, but certainly they are not our only sources. Many types of fish contain appreciable amounts of calcium as do most leafy vegetables. Whole wheat and rye flours contain more than white flour. Calcium is also easily obtainable in tablet form. Bone meal tablets or wafers sold in health food stores are an especially desirable way of building up the body's calcium intake.

R. What makes them so desirable?

A. Because research done in Sweden strongly suggests that bone meal offers protection against tooth decay as well. It is not just the calcium in the bone meal but some trace elements found along with it that seem to provide this particular benefit. However, if you start taking calcium supplements you should begin taking magnesium supplements too.

R. Why?

A. Because these two minerals seem to work together. The more you have of one, the more you should have of the other. And when it comes to coping with high blood pressure and its attendant ailments, magnesium may be even more important than calcium.

R. Why is this?

A. In the case of magnesium, we have some evidence directly linking it with HBP. In 1963, the *Journal of Applied Nutrition* reported research showing that animals made deficient in magnesium tended to develop hypertension. Two years later, the *Journal of the American Medical Association* noted that magnesium relaxed the walls of the arteries. As we saw in Chapter 1, the tensing or hardening of these walls can cause or catalyze high blood pressure. In 1976, Dr. Jean Mayer reported in his nationally syndicated newspaper column that monkeys fed high fat diets suffer much less hardening of the arteries if they are also fed plenty of magnesium. The same effect had earlier been noticed in rats.

R. I would suppose, then, that magnesium, like calcium, also tends to prevent heart disease?

A. If anything, it seems to outperform calcium in

this respect as well. For example studies in both England and Canada have shown that people living in hard water areas suffer substantially fewer heart attacks than those living in areas where the water is naturally soft. Both the calcium and magnesium which are found in much greater amounts in hard water than in soft were found to be responsible for this beneficial effect. However, when some medical researchers at the University of Toronto did some follow-up studies in their own province, they pinpointed the magnesium as the principal benefactor. As the research team's leader, Dr. T. W. Anderson, put it, "the higher cardiac death rate in the soft water areas of Ontario is due to the relative lack of magnesium in the water supply."

R. Has magnesium ever been used in the treatment of heart illness?

A. Two West German doctors have reported striking successes in giving both magnesium and potassium to heart patients. The two minerals are administered in the form of orotates. This means that they are put into a mineral base which helps transport them to the heart. In addition, one of them, Dr. Hans Nieper of Hanover, also gives his patients bromelain, an enzyme found in pineapple stems. This presumably helps his patients absorb and assimilate the two minerals.

Dr. Nieper says that he has administered the minerals to more than 150 heart patients over a two year period and that less than five per cent of them suffered heart attacks. Ordinarily, so he says, 24 to 30 per cent would have died from heart attacks during this time.

R. Are any American doctors using magnesium and potassium in such a way?

A. A few have started to do so. One of them is Dr. Gary F. Gordon who is president of the American Academy of Medical Preventrics. Dr. Gordon claims to have given these two minerals to 700 cardiac patients for two years, producing a dramatic relief of symptoms in 85 per cent of them. One third of this group had already suffered heart attacks but after the potassium and magnesium therapy, less than one per cent succumbed to a new heart attack.

R. In order to prevent heart problems from arising as well as to lower blood pressure, how much magnesium should we consume and how much do we consume?

A. The Food and Nutrition Board didn't even get around to setting a Recommended Dietary Allowance for magnesium until 1969. It put the figure at 350 milligrams for an adult but at 400 milligrams for young men. Many, including Dr. Mildred S. Seelig, who has done extensive research on magnesium—you may recall, she was quoted in Chapter 1 as noting that women seem to be able to metabolize or process magnesium better than men—feel that these figures are too low and 500 milligrams a day is a better goal to strive for.

However, the evidence indicates that most Americans fail to achieve even the amounts recommended by the Food and Nutrition Board. For example, a 1976 study of meals served to college students showed that these meals supplied only an average of 251 milligrams of magnesium a day. This was less than two-thirds of the amount needed to meet the minimum RDA requirement for young males.

R. Yes, but college students, like the rest of us, also snack between meals and after meals. Maybe in this way they were making up the difference.

A. It's more likely that such snacks would have the reverse effect. Sugar, for instance, tends to flush magnesium from the body. Alcohol, which is a form of sugar, will do the same. In 1971 a physician named Dr. John Prutting wrote in *Family Circle* magazine that "Seventy per cent of us have mismanaged our diets enough to have some degree of magnesium deficiency."

Meanwhile those people taking medication for hypertension may have the greatest problem of all in terms of magnesium.

R. Why is this?

A. Physicians frequently treat HBP by prescribing diuretics. As we saw earlier, these diuretics tend to flush out potassium and so to make up for this they will often prescribe potassium in supplemental form. The trouble is that the diuretics cause magnesium to be lost along with the potassium. This not only deprives the patient of a mineral valuable in its own right but it also renders the potassium supplements almost useless, for potassium can't do its job, indeed it can't even get to the cells of the body, without magnesium.

R. Why don't doctors, then, do something about this when they prescribe diuretics?

A. Few of them know about it. The research revealing this fact was published in the April 1, 1978 issue of the *British Medical Journal*. It has not, to my knowledge, been reported in any medical magazine in this country. One or two health magazines have cited the study but only a comparatively few doctors read such magazines. In the meantime, anyone taking diuretics should start taking steps to increase his or her intake of magnesium. For that matter, so should most of us.

R. How can we do this? What foods provide magnesium?

A. Magnesium is one of the more commonly found food minerals. Unfortunately, and unlike calcium, it is easily destroyed in processing. Whole wheat is quite rich in magnesium but 80 per cent of it will be lost when the grain is processed into white flour. Milk contains a fair amount of magnesium but much of it will be destroyed through pasteurization. (Magnesium is highly susceptible to heat.) Beans of various kinds, many vegetables and even shell fish contain magnesium. Nuts and seeds are especially abundant in this mineral. And besides whole wheat, there are oats and other whole grains.

Magnesium supplements are available in health food stores. Many of these come mixed with calcium on a two-for-one ratio. That is, the supplement will have twice as much calcium as magnesium. This is a good ratio since it is believed that the system should receive two to three times as much calcium as magnesium. Both can help lower your blood pressure and, more importantly perhaps, help protect you from the consequences which a higher-than-desirable blood pressure can produce.

R. So far you have mentioned only minerals that help. What about others like sodium that do harm?

A. We now move into the area of what are called trace minerals. We normally come into contact with only very minute amounts of these minerals yet these minute amounts can cause a great deal of mischief or benefit, as the case may be.

Most of the research regarding them is quite recent. It wasn't until the Dartmouth Medical School set up a trace mineral laboratory after World War II that scientists and research physicians began paying much attention to the role such minerals play in human health. But the discoveries of this laboratory, under the leadership of a physician named Henry A. Schroeder, have sparked interest among nutritional researchers everywhere. Most doctors, of course, know next to nothing about this research since, as we saw earlier, they almost seem to shield themselves from anything relating to nutrition. But those physicians, and remember that their numbers, while still few, are growing, who do concern themselves with the nutritional side of medicine, have welcomed and warmly endorsed the findings of Dr. Schroeder and his colleagues. Most of their discoveries have been substantiated and amplified by researchers elsewhere.

R. What discoveries have Dr. Schroeder and his group made concerning blood pressure?

A. They have found that a trace mineral called cadmium can send blood pressure shooting skyward. Rats exposed to small amounts of cadmium in their diet develop over their lifetime what Dr. Schroeder called "the full picture of human hypertension."

As for humans, Dr. Schroeder noted that the kidneys of Japanese people generally contain twice as much cadmium as those of Americans, while our kidneys, in turn, contain about four times as much cadmium as those of Africans. The high blood pressure rates follow the same pattern. There is more hypertension in Japan than in the U.S. and much more in the U.S. than in Africa.

Finally, in doing autopsies he and his collaborators found that those people who had suffered from HBP had much more cadmium in their bodies than those whose BP had been normal.

R. Where did all this cadmium come from?

A. Essentially from industrialization. Cadmium is used in many industrial processes and tiny amounts of it can enter the atmosphere. For example, cadmium is used as a stabilizer for rubber and sites near a highway are likely to have more cadmium in their air.

The phosphates we now use in chemical fertilizers may also contribute to the problem for some research suggests that they cause growing crops to absorb more cadmium. And our water supply is becoming prone to cadmium pollution. One survey of samples from 720 reservoirs and rivers used for drinking water found that 40 per cent of them contained cadmium.

Cadmium can also accumulate in water pipes so that it is a good practice to let the water flow for at least a few moments before using it. Dr. Schroeder even went so far as to urge people to draw their breakfast water the night before to avoid the overnight accumulations of cadmium.

R. Is there anything else we can do to protect ourselves from cadmium?

A. Fortunately, yes. Just as sodium has a natural enemy in potassium so cadmium has a natural enemy as well. Indeed it has three such enemies. One of them is another trace mineral: zinc.

R. You mean we should eat zinc?

A. We already do and people who are eating good diets are consuming appreciable amounts of it. Some zinc is required for normal health and the recommended daily allowance has been set at 15 milligrams. However, those concerned about cadmium, and that should include nearly all of us, should try to double that figure.

R. How much zinc is present in the average American diet?

A. Substantially less, it would appear, than the recommended daily allowance. Again, food processing is a major culprit. Just as whole wheat loses 80 per cent of its magnesium in being turned into white flour, so does it lose about the same proportion of its zinc as well.

There is also another factor which is reducing our zinc intake. The chemical fertilizers which are increasing the cadmium content of our crops are reducing their zinc content at the same time.

51

R. *I know that the health nuts have been making a big to-do about chemical fertilizers destroying or at least damaging the nutritional quality of our crops. But the government claims that fertilizers do not affect the nutritional level of crops and cites several studies to this effect. Don't you believe them?*

A. These studies are quite correct as far as they go. The trouble is they do not go far enough. It may be true that the type of fertilizer used to grow a crop will not directly affect the number and amount of nutrients in that crop. The key word here is "directly." What the fertilizer can and will do is affect the quality of the soil itself and soil quality in turn can greatly influence the trace minerals in the plant it produces.

The Food and Nutrition Board of the National Research Council has admitted this. In a statement issued in 1976, the Board spoke out against those who claim that chemical fertilizers affect plant quality. But at the same time, in the very same statement, it acknowledged that such fertilizers can seriously affect the number and amount of trace minerals in the soil. It also admitted that deficiencies of trace minerals in the soil can cause deficiencies of these same minerals in crops in that soil.

R. *Is there any real evidence that such fertilizers are making our crops deficient in zinc?*

A. The December, 1969 issue of *The National Hog Farmer* carried an article pointing out that the nation's pigs were starting to show surprisingly strong signs of suffering from severe stress. Some were even going into convulsions and dying. The two scientists who authored the article claimed that zinc deficiencies were causing this. The animals were being fed sweet corn grown with artificial fertilizers, they said, and this had caused the amount of zinc in the corn to sink to dangerous levels. Zinc, you should understand, has many more functions than simply that of combatting cadmium. Among these functions is providing protection against stress or against the effects of stress.

R. What about humans? Are we showing any signs of needing more zinc?

A. Not too many of us are suddenly going into convulsions and dying, but judging from all the books being written about it, we seem to be becoming increasingly more susceptible to stress. Many people blame this on the stress which is supposed to be inherent in our modern way of life. They overlook the fact that modern society has actually removed many of the sources of severe stress that characterized the lives of our forebears. I am referring to such modern developments as health insurance and unemployment insurance. Imagine the stress of struggling to support a family during the great depression of the 1930s!

Zinc has also been shown to be important to the proper functioning of the human immunization system and certainly we seem more prone to contracting certain illnesses that our immunization systems strive to protect us against such as the common cold. Zinc also has a great deal to do with male sexual development and in this connection we should note the increasing impotence being observed in young men and the increasing incidence of prostate problems in older men. Some research shows that prostate problems often improve under zinc supplementation.

R. So you blame all these problems on zinc deficiencies?

A. Not completely. Psychological factors may well be the major reason why so many young males today suffer from at least occasional impotence. Nevertheless, the current trends in human health in this country appear consistent with an insufficiency of zinc in the diet.

Certainly we could do much to improve our health generally as well as counteract the effects of all the cadmium around us by increasing our intake of zinc. As Dr. Schroeder observed, "An excess of zinc would prevent accumulation of cadmium while a slight deficiency [would] allow it."

R. How can we obtain this extra zinc?

A. Certain foods do contain substantial amounts of this vital trace mineral. The richest of them in this respect are oysters, especially those found on the Atlantic Coast. Pacific oysters have somewhat less although they still have a good deal. Another good and less expensive source are herrings and don't forget that sardines are herrings, too. Most meats also contain some zinc with liver being especially abundant in the mineral. Cheddar cheese is another good source.

When it comes to plant food, your best bets are wheat and other grains, provided they have not been processed. Three and a half ounces of wheat germ will fulfill the requirement of the recommended daily allowance. However, that would be quite a lot of wheat germ to consume in one day. Furthermore, as noted earlier, it would be wise to double the 15 milligrams called for by the RDA, especially if one is concerned about blood pressure.

R. Can one take zinc in supplemental form?

A. Yes. Zinc supplements are now available in most health food stores as well as some drug stores.

R. How much do you recommend that we take?

A. To obtain the excess which Dr. Schroeder called for, I would recommend 30 milligrams a day in supplement form regardless of how much may be in your daily diet. Many health oriented people, including some doctors, take even more than that.

R. You mentioned that cadmium had three natural enemies. What are the other two?

A. One of them has become the source of some of the most exciting developments on the scientific scene, at least as far as human health is concerned. This is a trace mineral called selenium.

R. Selenium? I must say I have never heard of this mineral before.

A. Regrettably neither have most doctors except, perhaps, for a slight brush with it while taking chemistry in pre-med school. But thanks to the pioneering work being done by biochemists on this mineral in recent years, some of the more health-oriented physicians are showing great interest. *Executive Health*, whose editorial board consists of some of the most eminent physicians and scientists in the country, published in March, 1979 a lengthy piece by one of the biochemists who has been investigating selenium.

R. What did he say?

A. The scientist, Dr. Raymond L. Shumberger of the Cleveland Clinic Foundation, spotlighted selenium's ability to neutralize the hypertensive effect of cadmium.

R. By effect you mean, I suppose, things like heart attacks and strokes?

A. Right. His research as well as that of others he cited showed, among other things, that those areas where selenium was present in the soil had substantially lower rates of such illnesses. Let me quote him directly.

"Americans living in selenium-poor areas are three times as likely to die from heart attacks, strokes, aneurysms (ballooning of the arteries due to weak artery walls), or other high blood pressure related causes, than are those residing in selenium rich areas of the country. Our epidemiologic study showed that people living in areas where selenium is found have a high blood pressure death rate of only one-third that of persons living in low selenium areas. We do not know selenium's precise action concerning high blood pressure but our study strongly suggests that it has a beneficial effect on high blood pressure problems in man, similar to that produced in laboratory animals at other research centers."

R. In other words, Dr. Shumberger's findings are based on laboratory studies with animals along with statistical studies in human beings?

A. He and his collaborators have gone even further. They have tested the blood found in representative blood banks in 19 states. They found that those blood samples from states showing high rates of hypertension and heart disease contained much less selenium than those from states where the incidence of such illness was low.

R. What are the so-called high blood pressure states?

A. They include Connecticut, Illinois, Ohio, Oregon, Massachusetts, Rhode Island, New York, Pennsylvania, Indiana and Delaware. The soil in these states tends to have little or no selenium and the high blood pressure rate ranges up to 300 per cent higher than in the selenium-rich states.

R. What are the selenium-rich states?

A. They include Texas, Oklahoma, Arizona, Colorado, Louisiana, Utah, Alabama, Nebraska, Kansas, North and South Dakota. The high blood pressure death rate is comparatively low in all these states.

R. So their inhabitants don't have to worry about getting enough selenium.

A. I don't think Dr. Shumberger and the other scientists who have investigated selenium would say that. Their conclusion seems to be that nearly all of us could benefit from an increased intake of selenium.

R. How can we obtain this additional selenium?

A. Some foods contain much more of it than others.

Whole wheat flour has nearly four times as much selenium as white flour. Oats also supply selenium and the commercial oat cereal called Cheerios provides a fair amount of this mineral. Rice is a good provider of selenium and so are eggs. For example egg noodles, even when made from white flour, constitute one of the best sources of selenium in the diet. Sesame seeds and brewers yeast are prime sources of selenium.

R. *What about meat and fish?*

A. Many kinds of fish contain a good deal of it. Shellfish are perhaps foremost in this respect. Unfortunately, most of them are also high in cadmium and sodium. But other kinds of fish also contain selenium. These include swordfish, cod and tuna.

Meat generally has little selenium but there are exceptions. Liver has some while kidneys have much more.

R. *And vegetables?*

A. Also not generally a good source but again there are exceptions. Garlic supplies some selenium; mushrooms somewhat less.

Selenium is also now available in supplement form. One has to exercise some caution in consuming such supplements, since this mineral can prove toxic if taken in large amounts. However, these tablets customarily contain only small amounts of selenium and as long as one does not exceed the recommended dosages he or she should encounter no danger. However, a proper diet stressing the selenium-rich foods cited above should give most of us all the selenium we need.

R. So selenium joins zinc as a natural antagonist to cadmium?

A. Yes, but one should not look upon them as simply counter-active agents for cadmium. They both have much more positive roles to play in preserving and protecting health. They would be of value even if there were no cadmium in our environment. The same holds true for the third natural enemy to cadmium. This is chromium.

R. I thought chromium was something we used to plate car fenders or bumpers with. You mean it's something that's good for us to eat?

A. Yes. Dr. Schroeder found that it helped protect laboratory animals against atherosclerosis and also extended their life span. Rats given chromium supplements lived for four years, setting a new record, he said, in longevity for this animal. He also found that chromium improved the body's ability to tolerate glucose (sugar) and therefore could prove most helpful to diabetics. Dr. Shumberger believes that its ability to increase glucose tolerance may account for the fact that people with high blood pressure tend to have low levels of chromium in their bodies.

R. I don't understand.

A. Well, people with low chromium levels appear to be more susceptible to diabetes and diabetics tend to be more susceptible to high blood pressure. In any case, we do know that those who suffer from high blood pressure tend to have less chromium in their bodies than those who do not, and this, together with its demonstrated advantageous effects on the arteries and life spans of experimental animals, should make us all conscious of consuming enough chromium.

R. How does one go about doing this?

A. Chromium in supplemental form has recently become available and such supplements are sold in many health food stores and some drug stores. Brewers yeast, liver, fruits and fruit juices are among the best sources of chromium in our daily diets. And once again, whole grains, including bran, will also supply appreciable amounts.

I should point out, that processed grains not only fail to supply adequate amounts of chromium but actually tend to destroy it. Dr. Schroeder found that white flour would gradually cause the body to lose chromium over the years. He found that white sugar would do this even more. But honey and molasses, on the other hand, would tend to add to the body's supplies of chromium. Even dark brown sugar would do so provided the sugar was so brown that it would stick together. So we see that with grains and sugars, processing not only makes them chromium deficient but actually chromium destructive. By the way, it should be noted that white sugar may also have a negative effect on zinc, that is it may tend to destroy or drive out our system's minute but important supplies of this mineral as well.

R. Judging from what you have said so far, some foods tend to be naturally rich in nearly all of the substances that lower blood pressure or at least curb some of its more harmful effects. Fruits, vegetables, whole grains and fish seem generally to be the good

guys, while meat, processed grains and sugar come out looking pretty badly.

A. That may be oversimplifying things a bit. Some meats, especially organ meats such as liver and kidney, not only have favorable potassium to sodium ratios, but also contain appreciable amounts of zinc, selenium and other valuable trace minerals. On the other hand, some fish, such as crabs and oysters, are naturally quite high in sodium. But certainly a diet rich in fruits, vegetables and whole grains and low in processed grains and sugar can help greatly in curbing high blood pressure and in fostering good health generally.

CHAPTER 4

What Vitamins Can Do

R. A lot of hoopla is being made these days by the so called health nuts about vitamins. I recognize that vitamins are essential to life but the American Dietetic Association and the American Medical Association maintain that we get all the vitamins we need from a well-balanced diet. I trust that you agree.

A. No, I do not agree at all.

R. Don't you think you are being foolish in challenging such organizations as those I have mentioned? What gives you the right to think that you know more than they do?

A. What gives me the right to do so is the fact that many of the most distinguished medical researchers in the world also appear to disagree with their position.

R. Who are these researchers?

A. They include at least three Nobel prize winners in medicine, Dr. Albert Szent-Gyorgyi, Dr. Linus Pauling and Dr. Hans Krebs. Dr. Pauling, by the way, is the only person ever to win two unshared Nobel prizes.

Other apparent dissenters include Dr. Alton Ochsner, the dean of American heart surgeons and founder of the famed Ochsner Clinic and hospital in New Orleans; Dr. Charles Butterworth, a professor of medicine at the University of Alabama and a former chairman of the AMA's own food and nutrition committee; Dr. Arthur Upton, former head of the National Cancer Institute; and even Dr. Theodore Cooper who, as former Assistant Secretary for Health for the Department of Health, Education and Welfare, can be considered, in a sense, the nation's former top doctor. I could cite others as, or almost as, distinguished as these I have just mentioned who apparently disagree with the stand that no one needs more vitamins than those available in the so-called well-balanced diet.

R. Why do you keep qualifying what you say with the words "apparent" or "apparently"?

A. Because, except for Dr. Pauling, none of them have directly challenged the position espoused by the American Dietetic Association or the AMA. Yet, every single one of them is on record as saying that they take extra vitamins themselves and/or recommend the taking of such vitamins to their patients. And let me repeat that they are only a few of the highly regarded medical men and women who have signified their belief in the utility of taking extra vitamins. Thus, anyone who takes vitamin pills will find himself in mighty good company.

R. On what basis do these medical men you mentioned endorse the taking of extra vitamins?

A. On the basis of a mounting accumulation of evidence that pretty much proves that vitamin dosages beyond the low RDA's (Recommended Dietary Allowances) can improve human health as well as alleviate many medical problems. Among these problems are those related to high blood pressure.

R. Just what can vitamins do to lower blood pressure?

A. I did not say lower it but relieve or reduce certain problems related to it. Keeping that in mind, they can be most useful.

Let's start by examining vitamin C.

As far back as 1953, two research physicians reported in the magazine *Geriatrics* on a four-year experiment in which they gave varying amounts of vitamin C to 32 elderly patients all of whom were suffering from vascular disease (problems with their blood vessels). During the entire four years only six or less than one-fifth of these patients died. That in itself was something of a medical miracle considering the age and condition of these people. Of the six who did die, four, predictably enough, died from heart attacks. But what was especially interesting was that these four had belonged to *the group who had been receiving the smallest amounts of vitamin C.*

The following year, two California physicians reported on a seven-year study. They had randomly selected 577 people who were 50 years old or older and questioned them closely on their food intake. Then in tracking them over the next seven years, they found that those whose diets were the most abundant in vitamin C had a much lower death rate than those whose diets contained less of the vitamin. Most of the deaths with this group, as with the population at large, were from cardiovascular disease. Meanwhile, in that same year the *Canadian Medical Association Journal* carried a research report which showed that hardening arteries contain less vitamin C than arteries not afflicted by this problem.

In 1966 a doctor named Boris Sokoloff reported in the *Journal of the American Geriatrics Society* that he had seen "improvement ranging from moderate to impressive" in 50 out of 60 patients suffering from atherosclerosis following administration of 1,000 to 3,000 milligrams of vitamin C a day. Please keep in mind that atherosclerosis and arteriosclerosis can both produce high blood pressure.

R. Is this the evidence that impressed some of the doctors you cited earlier?

A. Yes. Dr. Butterworth and one of his colleagues wrote an article in *The American Journal of Clinical Nutrition* in 1974 in which they said that "A rather large volume of literature supports the hypothesis that vitamin C decreases susceptibility to vascular injury..." They also pointed to research showing vitamin C to be helpful in preventing and, in its early stages, even reversing hardening of the arteries. In 1978, Dr. Alton Ochsner wrote an article for *Executive Health* entitled "On the Role of Vitamins C and E in Medicine." He also reviewed and endorsed this and other research supporting vitamin C's utility in this area of concern.

R. How much vitamin C does one need to gain these benefits?

A. Dr. Butterworth and his colleagues believe 900 milligrams a day is the *minimum* needed for good health. He says that one can take up to 2,000 a day with no fear of any negative consequences. Other doctors place the safe and desirable level much higher. Dr. Robert Cathcart, in an address to the California Orthomolecular Medical Association in 1978, said that everyone should take vitamin C up to the point of getting diarrhea. When that point is reached, they should cut back to an amount just below it. Until you get diarrhea, he said, you are not taking too much vitamin C.

R. And who is this Dr. Cathcart? He sounds like something of a nut.

A. He was one of the most respected orthopedic surgeons in the country. The Cathcart prothesis, which he invented, is widely used by orthopedists everywhere. However, I say "was" because a few years ago he became so excited over the possibilities of using nutrition and other new approaches in medicine that he gave up orthopedics for general practice. He is one of the growing number of doctors who have taken the time and trouble to follow the developments in these fields and who have changed their ideas and practice accordingly.

R. How do I get all this vitamin C? By drinking orange juice?

A. Orange juice is certainly a good natural source of vitamin C. So are other citrus fruits as well as many vegetables. But to obtain even the minimum amounts which Dr. Butterworth recommends, that is 1,000 to 2,000 milligrams a day, you will probably have to take the vitamin in tablet form. It takes 10 full glasses of fresh or frozen orange juice to provide 1,000 milligrams of vitamin C.

R. Is the vitamin C that comes in tablet form as good as the vitamin C which nature provides?

A. For the most part, yes. Vitamin C is simply another name for a chemical known as ascorbic acid, and it can be manufactured quite easily and cheaply. However, some rather interesting related substances are often found with vitamin C in its natural state and most synthetic preparations of the vitamin fail to include them.

R. What are these substances and what, if anything, are they good for?

A. They are called the bioflavonoids. The Food and Nutrition Board claims that the bioflavonoids have no proven value to the human system but many researchers disagree. Dr. Szent-Gyorgyi, who won the Nobel prize in the 1930s for discovering vitamin C, has continually insisted that the bioflavonoids improve the functioning of the capillaries and at least some research now exists to support his claim.

Dr. B. F. Hart, a Fort Lauderdale, Florida physician who has done extensive work with vitamin C, agrees with Dr. Szent-Gyorgyi. Dr. Hart says that the bioflavonoids are especially important to people with high blood pressure or diabetes since such patients tend to have fragile capillaries which makes them prone to stroke and other medical problems. "In some of these people," he writes, "there are small areas of ruptured blood vessels in the brain that lead to progressive mental deterioration. The other trouble areas are in the coronary vessels of the heart. There are found tiny capillary hemorrhages, the forerunner of blood clots. For the above reasons, I recommend that my patients in these categories eat raw fruits and take currently available bioflavonoids."

R. What about people who do not have diabetes and who don't even have high blood pressure as it is normally defined? Does it pay for them to take bioflavonoids, too?

A. Yes. They appear to be useful to us all. Dr. Emanuel Cheraskin, a professor of medicine at the University of Alabama and the author of some 13 books on nutrition, recommends their consumption. So do Dr. Carlton Fredericks, a former president of the International Academy of Preventive Medicine, and a host of others.

R. Can you buy bioflavonoid tablets?

A. Yes, they are available in health food stores, sometimes as part of vitamin C preparations but also separately as well. While fresh fruits are the most common source of the bioflavonoids in nature, buckwheat also contains goodly amounts of them.

R. What about vitamin E? I notice that the article you cited by Dr. Ochsner was entitled "On the Role of Vitamins C and E in Medicine." Does Dr. Ochsner believe in taking vitamin E as well as vitamin C?

A. In his article he mentions that he has been routinely prescribing vitamin E to all patients who seem prone to blood clots in their veins. He has been doing this for over 30 years with good results. A good deal of research now exists to back him up. For example, at a conference on vitamin E in 1973, several studies came to light showing that the vitamin improves circulation in the legs and arms. It apparently alleviates arteriosclerosis in these organs and any substance that does that is likely to have a beneficial effect on blood pressure as well.

R. So far, so good. But is that all vitamin E can do to affect blood pressure?

A. The vitamin seems to improve the general functioning of the heart. By 1942, only a few years after the vitamin was discovered, two researchers reported in the *Journal of Biological Chemistry* that the heart muscles needed less oxygen to function properly when vitamin E had been supplied. Administration of the vitamin could reduce the amount of required oxygen by as much as 42 per cent.

In the mid 1950s, new research showed that test animals made deficient in vitamin E quickly became vulnerable to all kinds of heart and arterial problems. On the positive side, supplying extra vitamin E tended to dilate (enlarge) their blood vessels and make them more resistant to induced heart attacks. In his book *Nutrition Against Disease*, Dr. Roger J. Williams cites this research as supporting the claim that vitamin E "opens up blood vessels and thus salvages heart attack victims." Don't forget that anything that opens up blood vessels will tend to lower blood pressure or at least will help prevent it from going higher.

R. Who is Dr. Roger J. Williams, by the way?

A. He is probably America's most distinguished biochemist, the first biochemist to be elected president of the American Chemistry Society. He discovered an important B vitamin called pantothenic acid and discovered a good deal of information about another B vitamin called folic acid. He himself used to suffer angina pains but appears to have gotten rid of them through taking certain vitamins, among them vitamin E.

R. Where does one find vitamin E?

A. Whole wheat flour, oatmeal, brown rice, unprocessed vegetable oils and green vegetables are some of the best natural sources. But as with vitamin C, it is usually necessary to take it in tablet form in order to obtain the amounts necessary for maximum benefit.

R. How much vitamin E should one take?

A. That depends. Dr. Evan Shute, a Canadian cardiologist who used the vitamin extensively in his practice, recommended 600 units a day for the average woman and 800 units for the average man. For older people and those with heart problems, he urged and used much larger amounts. He himself took 2,400 units a day. Linus Pauling currently takes 1,600 units while Dr. Lawrence Steiner, a blood research specialist and professor of medicine at Brown University, says he takes 1,200 units a day. There is one caveat or cautionary note, however.

R. What is that?

A. Although the vitamin appears to be advantageous to those wishing to keep their BP low, large amounts can *temporarily* cause an elevation in blood pressure in *some* people. Those who already suffer from high blood pressure should start slowly with perhaps only 90 units a day for a month. They can then gradually increase the dosage and eventually they will reap the benefits which the vitamin can bestow.

R. So much for vitamins C and E. What about the others?

A. As you perhaps know, there is no one B vitamin but a whole group of vitamins known as the B complex. Some of these can help greatly in the fight against HBP and its consequences.

Let's start with vitamin B6 or pyridoxine. Dr. Williams, whom I quoted earlier, lists in his book a host of well-controlled, scientific experiments indicating "very strongly that vitamin B6 is another key element" in the control of high blood pressure and blood vessel problems. High blood pressure can be easily induced in laboratory rats by feeding them diets deficient in this vitamin. Atherosclerotic tissue has been found to contain lower levels of B6 than normal tissue with the difference being especially pronounced in males. Also feeding monkeys extra B6 reduces their cholesterol levels.

R. I note that many of these experiments had to do with an actual deficiency in B6. How common are such deficiencies?

A. Very common, according to Dr. Williams. The recommended dietary allowance has been set at only two milligrams a day but most Americans, he says, don't even receive this much through the daily diet. B6, so it seems, is quite unstable and is therefore easily destroyed by heat and other forms of food processing. Also, Dr. Williams feels that two milligrams is far below the amount desirable for daily consumption.

R. Where do we get B6?

A. Meats, especially organ meats such as liver, as well as fish supply it. So do whole grains, nuts and seeds. Bananas are another good source. But, here again, anyone who wishes to make maximum use of the vitamin should take 50 milligrams of it in tablet form, preferably twice a day.

R. What about other B vitamins?

A. Dr. Williams also has high regard for choline in this connection. Choline is a member of the B complex group but is not in itself an official vitamin. I mean that the Food and Nutrition Board has not deemed it necessary to human health. Yet experiments, some of them going back a long time, show it to have potentially great significance for many medical problems including HBP.

Experiments reported in 1949 showed that animals would get HBP from diets in which choline was lacking. In 1957, a remarkable experiment involving 158 patients was reported. All of these patients had dangerously high blood pressure but every single one of them experienced a drop in blood pressure after being given choline supplements daily for a period of three weeks. In over a third, blood pressure actually fell to normal levels.

R. Can choline be found in tablet form?

A. Better stocked health stores carry it. The best foods for choline are brewers yeast, eggs, fish, soybeans, peanuts and liver.

R. What about the other B vitamins?

A. Well, niacin, which is B3, tends to dilate the arteries. In causing the walls of the arteries to expand and thus allowing blood to pour through these vessels more easily, it can reduce blood pressure. Unfortunately, the effect is not permanent. Still, taken regularly, perhaps at every meal, it could prove helpful.

Another advantageous aspect of niacin lies in its effect on cholesterol. I have not said much about the cholesterol question so far since it is quite complex and controversial. However, high amounts of certain kinds of cholesterol in the blood are associated with atherosclerosis or fatty deposits on the walls of the arteries and this situation, as we saw in Chapter 1, can narrow the passageways, thereby forcing the heart to work harder and causing an attendant rise in blood pressure. Consequently, a cholesterol problem can produce or aggravate a blood pressure problem.

In 1956 the world-famed Mayo Clinic reported the results of giving high doses of niacin (3,000 milligrams a day) to 13 high cholesterol patients for 12 weeks. Nine of the 13 or nearly three-quarters of them experienced a significant drop in cholesterol level. Several other studies were reported the following year showing similar results. Some of them were described in the *Canadian Medical Association Journal* of December 15, 1957.

However, some side effects did seem to result from taking such heavy dosages of this vitamin. They included facial flushing, some irritation of the intestinal tract and, in certain patients, signs of possible liver malfunctioning. But taken in smaller amounts, say up to 500 milligrams twice a day, niacin could still produce some benefits while at the same time not producing any problems.

R. Are there any other B vitamins that are helpful?

A. Folic acid also appears to be of some importance in circulatory regulation. The offspring of laboratory animals fed diets deficient in this B vitamin tend to have malformed hearts and blood vessels. The same consequences have also been observed in the offspring of animals who have been made deficient in vitamin A.

R. What about taking extra amounts of vitamin A? Will that assist us in lowering blood pressure?

A. There is no evidence that it will. But it is a valuable vitamin. Furthermore, one of its best sources may greatly aid us in cholesterol control.

R. What do you mean?

A. I mean cod liver oil which is a prime source of vitamin A. Some recent research has shown cod liver oil to have other uses as well.

A group of Danish scientists became intrigued by the fact that Greenland Eskimos have low cholesterol levels and other favorable patterns of heart health including moderate blood pressure. Yet these Eskimos consume huge quantities of animal fat. In 1978, the researchers reported finding the answer in a fatty acid called EPA. (It's real name is eicosapentaenioc acid, a jaw-breaker for even scientists to pronounce.) EPA, said the Danish scientists, helps prevent blood clots and deposits on the arterial walls.

Now, it appears that EPA is found most abundantly in certain types of Arctic fish, and the Eskimos, in consuming such fish as part of their daily diet, managed to keep themselves remarkably free of heart and circulatory ailments. The lesson here is obvious: eat plenty of cod. Try to take some cod liver oil, too. It's obtainable in tablet form if you don't like the taste of the oil.

R. You seem to have pretty much covered the waterfront as far as vitamins are concerned. Apparently just about all of them help control blood pressure.

A. Not really. For one thing, I did leave out some of the B vitamins as well as vitamin D. Furthermore, many of those I did cite only help blood pressure regulation indirectly, most often by helping to ward off arterial problems. But all the vitamins are essential to human health and this, after all, is our basic goal. So be sure to get enough of them all and enjoy more fully the longer life which a lowered blood pressure, as well as good health generally, should provide.

CHAPTER 5

Foods: The Good and the Bad

R. You have already pointed up the value of fruits, vegetables, whole grains, some kinds of fish and liver as suppliers of various vitamins and minerals that aid blood pressure control. Is there anything else to consider in the nutrition department?

A. Yes, there is. Some foods and food substances, in addition to the ones we have examined, seem to have a special impact, positive or negative as the case may be, on blood pressure.

R. What are they?

A. Let's begin by looking at those which benefit blood pressure control. There are a good many of them but the one I would put at the top of the list is garlic.

R. Garlic? I've heard garlic mentioned occasionally from time to time as having some sort of special powers but I thought that was just folklore.

Renaissance Bookstore

230
Hamilton Avenue
Palo Alto, CA
94301

415.321.2846

MON-SAT
10 AM - 9 PM

SUNDAY
12 PM - 6 PM

We Buy, Sell & Trade
Quality Books & Records.
Phone for buying hours.

A. Never make fun of folklore, at least when it comes to health. Every day evidence turns up showing that what was thought to be a popular superstition has been found to be partly or wholly true. Such appears to have been the case with garlic.

Reports by doctors who succeeded in lowering blood pressure in animals or humans by feeding them garlic began appearing in European medical journals almost 60 years ago. One of the more authoritative of these reports was published in 1948. A Swiss physician who was also a professor of medicine at the University of Geneva told of treating 100 patients with garlic. He had them consume large amounts of it for a few weeks but then allowed them to taper off.

He claimed that the garlic significantly lowered the blood pressure in 40 per cent of these patients with the results starting to show after only a week. He took every precaution to see to it that the reduction in BP was due to the garlic they consumed and nothing else.

The drop in blood pressure was accompanied by other favorable developments. HBP symptoms such as dizziness disappeared. What's more, almost all of them, including those whose blood pressure did not go down, claimed they could think more clearly. This may seem surprising but there have been other indications that garlic can do this. For example, Eleanor Roosevelt ate three garlic balls dipped in chocolate every day, claiming that they helped keep her mentally alert.

R. A 40 per cent reduction is impressive but nevertheless it means that the majority were not helped. Also, the experiment does not seem to have been subject to strict scientific controls such as the use of a comparison group of similar patients who did not re-

ceive the garlic and the use of outside evaluators to tabulate the results.

A. True on both counts. As for the lack of strict scientific controls, we should note that the results do coincide with that of earlier experiments and with the experience of numerous individuals. Health magazines over the years have received letters from many persons claiming that garlic has helped them lower their blood pressure. But, again, it does not work for everyone.

Concerning your other point, may I say that if only 40 per cent of those taking garlic for this purpose should experience a significant decline in BP, then all or nearly all of them should benefit in other ways.

R. How so?

A. Garlic also has been found to have a remarkable ability to assist fat metabolism and thereby reduce cholesterol. It also helps in blood coagulation and in so doing it reduces the risk of strokes. Research on these points was published in the *Lancet* in 1973 and in 1975. Garlic has even been shown to assist the body's handling of sugar and thereby to be of aid in alleviating diabetes, an ailment that may not be unrelated to high blood pressure, for those who suffer from one of these conditions have an above average chance of suffering from the other. Science, in short, is tending to support age-old superstition regarding the healthful properties of this flavorful plant.

R. Garlic may be flavorful and healthy but it's also pretty smelly. Can't it be as harmful socially as it is helpful physically?

A. It doesn't have to be. The bad breath which comes from garlic can be greatly reduced if not eliminated by eating some parsley along with it. As a matter of fact, parsley will do double duty for not only does it tend to counteract garlic's odor but it also supplies a lot of valuable potassium. Also garlic can be consumed in tablet form. Health food stores sell what are called garlic perles and these do not cause appreciable mouth odor.

R. If garlic is as successful as you say in alleviating high blood pressure, helping the body process fats and acting as an anticoagulant, then I would suppose that countries which consume large amounts of it suffer lower rates of these medical maladies.

A. You suppose correctly. The heart attack rate in Italy is only one-third that of the United States. All through Southern Europe where garlic is extensively used there are lower incidences of heart disease and other high blood pressure problems. Of course, the people of these countries also tend to consume more potassium-rich fruits and vegetables, and to rely more on other spices besides just salt, than their Northern neighbors. These practices, which are at least partially continued by their descendants in this country, may well account for the blood pressure differences between darker-skin Whites and lighter-skin Whites that we noted in Chapter 1.

R. Onions seem related to garlic. At least they tend to produce bad breath. Do they tend to lower blood pressure as well?

A. I do not know of any evidence that they actually

lower BP but I have heard that they may have a slight impact in this direction. What I do know is that onions, like garlic, will help fat metabolism. In one experiment, human volunteers were fed large amounts of butter fat which elevated their cholesterol. Some were then fed onions while others were not. Those who ingested the onions found their cholesterol levels returning to normal, while the levels of those not receiving the onions were still rising.

Like garlic, onions also tend to increase the breakdown of fibrin, a substance needed for blood clotting.

R. But doesn't this pose danger? After all, if our blood did not clot we could bleed to death from a small cut.

A. Garlic and onions tend to reduce the fibrin just enough to help prevent unneeded and undesirable clotting. In so doing they allow the heart to pump the blood through the vessels more easily and with less pressure. But the research published on this in *Nutrition Reviews* of 1976 indicates that they do not interrupt or impair the blood's normal clotting action.

R. Chalk up one for folklore. Does such folk wisdom have any other foods to offer us in the search for lower blood pressure?

A. Yes. As you know, folklore has often leaned heavily on herbs and now science seems to be lending support to some of these claims. Take ginseng for example. It has long enjoyed a place of high esteem in Oriental health lore. Now, research has appeared showing such esteem to be based on fact. The Soviets have an institute in Vladivostok, near the Manchurian border, which has been carrying out extensive experiments with ginseng. In 1965, the institute's director, a Dr. I. I. Brekhman, announced finding that ginseng "normalized the level of arterial pressure" and had proven effective in treating both high and low blood pressure.

I would, however, warn you to be wary about using ginseng.

R. Why? Are there serious side effects? Or don't you believe what the Soviets say?

A. My hesitations about ginseng concern only the quality of the herb that is currently available. Ginseng is an unusual plant. It exhausts the soil in which it is grown so completely that another six or seven years are needed before a fresh crop can be harvested from the same soil. But due to the rising demand for ginseng, many Asian growers are planting crops every two or three years. You do not get effective ginseng that way. As I have said, it is a remarkable herb with many health giving properties, but, unless you choose to grow your own or have some assurances regarding the quality of what you buy, I hesitate recommending it.

R. Are there any other more accessible herbs that can help high blood pressure?

A. Numerous ones have been used for this purpose. At one time rural doctors in the U.S. used sassafras tea to treat HBP. George Zofehak, a chiropractor, recommends one-half teaspoon of valerian in a cup of water. He says the mixture should not be drunk all at once but sipped during the day. Maurice Mességué also has an herbal prescription for high blood pressure. Mességué is a well known French herbologist who has treated

European celebrities including the late Winston Churchill. Mességué considers garlic to be the strongest natural medicine for HBP but also cites hawthorn and lavender as useful. His prescription is as follows:

> 2 pinches of hawthorn flowers
> 1 pinch of lavender
> 5 grams (a little less than one-fifth of an ounce) of garlic

These should be steeped in a quart of water and drunk at the rate of two cups a day.

R. Are there any modern, bona fide physicians using herbs for high blood pressure?

A. Quite a few. One of them is Dr. Howard Posner, a former chief of the Infectious Disease Division at Lincoln Hospital in New York City and a former faculty member at the Albert Einstein Medical School. Like the orthopedic surgeon Dr. Cathcart, whom I cited in the previous chapter, Dr. Posner has become so excited about the possibilities of using nutrition and other natural methods for building health that he has abandoned his field of specialization for general practice.

The June, 1978 issue of *Prevention* carried an article about him. In it he was quoted as saying "I saw a woman with high blood pressure whose doctor had given her a strong, new medicine. It didn't work; she still had the high blood pressure and now she had side effects from the medicine, too! I stopped the medicine and told her to take an herbal drink of fennel, caraway, anise, mint, yarrow and chamomile three times a day. In 10 days she had no high blood pressure, and she looked much better."

R. So hawthorn, lavender, valerian, fennel, car-

away, anise, mint, yarrow and chamomile have all been used to treat high blood pressure! Where can I get such herbs? And which ones should I use and in what quantities?

A. Health food stores usually stock many of them, sometimes in combination or, most often, separately. You will probably find neither Dr. Posner's nor Mességué's recipe already prepared for consumption. But start experimenting with some of the teas that contain one or more of the herbs that have been mentioned. You may be pleasantly surprised not just by the effect they may have on your blood pressure but by the other beneficial consequences which they may produce.

R. Are there any other foods that belong on the lower-your-blood-pressure list?

A. Whey is at least a candidate for this list, and a formidable one at that.

R. Whey? You mean the stuff that Little Miss Muffet was eating in the nursery rhyme?

A. Yes. A nutrition writer named Linda Clark claims to have come across a study done by two physicians in a California State Prison in the early 1930s. She says the two doctors gave a rounded tablespoon of powdered whey, dissolved in water, to two groups of hypertensive inmates three times a day. Within three months the average systolic (top) blood pressure level fell from 180 to 148 in one group. In the second group the average systolic reading dropped from 194 to 163 in just 20 days.

I have not seen the study Clark mentions and she

does not document its source. Whey is believed to be an excellent food. It is consumed heavily, for instance, in that region in Southern Russia which has become famous for having so many oldsters that are over 100 years of age.

R. Just what is whey and where can it be obtained?

A. Whey is a derivative of milk and every dairy produces it. It could be easily and cheaply obtainable if there was a sizable demand for it. Since there is not such demand, it is usually thrown away. You might say that to the average dairyman, whey is a junk food. However, some health food stores do stock it.

R. Any other foods that are good for HBP?

A. None others that I know of. However, there are some foods, in addition to garlic and onions, which tend to lower cholesterol and to the extent that cholesterol may influence blood pressure, these foods can be expected to help bring it down. They are eggplant, alfalfa seeds, yogurt, plus foods containing pectin and foods containing lecithin (pronounced less-i-thin).

R. But cardiologists don't usually tell their patients to eat these foods to lower cholesterol. What evidence do you have that such foods actually do what you say they do?

A. An Austrian scientist, Dr. G. H. Mitschek of the University of Graz, has succeeded in countering the effects of cholesterol-producing diet fed to laboratory animals by feeding them supplemental amounts of eggplant. The eggplant, so he has reported, seemed to bind up the cholesterol and carry it out of their systems. We also know that those countries where eggplant is a popular food are countries where cholesterol problems are almost non-existent.

Dr. George V. Mann, the research physician from Vanderbilt University that I mentioned earlier, made the discovery regarding yogurt. He was doing some experiments among the milk-drinking Maseai tribe in Africa when he accidentally came across the yogurt-low cholesterol relationship. Back in this country he succeeded in lowering the cholesterol levels of a group of students by feeding them yogurt. Unfortunately, however, it takes fairly sizable quantities of yogurt to have an appreciable effect.

As for alfalfa, a team of scientists led by Dr. M. R. Malinow found they could feed monkeys an atherosclerosis-producing diet and yet protect them from getting atherosclerosis by feeding them alfalfa seeds along with it. Another group of monkeys which received the same diet but without the seeds developed, for the most part, atherosclerotic conditions. This research was carried out at the Oregon Regional Primate Research Center in Beaverton, Oregon. It should be pointed out, however, that all seeds contain copious amounts of fiber and this could have been the protective factor in this experiment.

R. What about pectin and lecithin? I haven't the vaguest idea what those substances are.

A. Pectin is found in most fruits, with the apple being perhaps the best source. Experiments at Rutgers University in New Jersey have revealed its cholesterol-lowering effect. However, I should point out that with both apples and alfalfa, as with yogurt, a goodly amount must be consumed before significant effects are noticed.

With apples, you would really need to eat two pounds a day. Happily pectin can be obtained in more concentrated forms and therefore can be consumed in copious amounts without having to eat pounds and pounds of apples. (Although apples in themselves are an excellent food.)

Experiments with lecithin go back to the early 1940s. They have shown that this fat-emulsifying substance does tend to lower blood cholesterol levels. For many years those doctors and nutritionists who deigned to even acknowledge these experiments insisted that they were inadequate to prove its cholesterol-lowering properties.

But in the 1970s, lecithin gained an increasing number of supporters including two distinguished ones, Dr. Roger Williams and Dr. Charles Butterworth, both of whom I have cited earlier in other connections.

Dr. Williams in his valuable book *Nutrition Against Disease* reviewed these experiments with lecithin and found them convincing. "Lecithin is an enemy of cholesterol deposits and consuming more lecithin is a useful preventive measure," he concluded. Incidentally, Dr. Williams' book is available in paperback and anyone interested in the problems we are discussing should read it, especially Chapter Five. Be sure also to read the notes for this chapter, which are found in the back of the book.

As for Dr. Butterworth, his endorsement of lecithin came in his 1974 article in which, as I mentioned earlier, he also endorsed vitamin C as a preventive of hardening of the arteries. Don't forget that Dr. Butterworth, in addition to being a professor of medicine at the University of Alabama, is also a former chairman of the Food and Nutrition Council of the American Medical Association.

R. *What foods contain lecithin?*

A. Eggs are the richest source. Soybeans probably come second. Lecithin can also be purchased in capsule, liquid or granular form at health food stores. The granular form, mixed in with other foods such as breakfast cereal, soups, etc. seems to work best.

R. *There certainly seems to be a lot of foods and food substances to alleviate high blood pressure and many of its related problems. When it comes to the bad guys in the food department, is the list as long?*

A. Fortunately, no. In addition to salt, which has already been covered, there are only three groups of foods which need to be avoided or at least minimized in the diet: sugar, some kinds of meat, refined carbohydrates and certain preservatives.

R. *Sugar? I have heard a lot of bad things about sugar and its effect on human health but I have never heard it cited as a contributor to high blood pressure. How does it do this?*

A. In many ways. First sugar consumption almost always leads to increased weight and increased weight almost always raises blood pressure. We shall be looking at this problem more closely later on. Then, sugar tends to promote stress which in turn tends to promote HBP.

R. *Promote stress? How?*

A. As you may know, sugar causes the pancreas to

pump out insulin to convert the sugar into a form that the body can absorb. But the pure, refined sugar we use today acts as too powerful a stimulant to the pancreas. As a result, the pancreas pumps out more insulin than the body needs. The ironic and seemingly contradictory result is actually a low level of sugar in the blood. Low blood sugar puts a good deal of stress on the system, making us feel irritable and restless.

R. You mean eating sugar gives us low blood sugar?

A. It tends to. Think of it in terms of a fire. If you put some crumpled papers on a slow-burning fire, you will get large flames and intense heat—for a few seconds. Then the fire will sink back to its formerly low level. Something akin to this happens when we eat refined sugar except the effect is more severe. Thanks to the over-supply of insulin which the sugar generates, the level of sugar in the blood ends up sinking lower than it was before. And this condition can and often will produce a certain amount of stress.

R. Does sugar have any other ill effects?

A. Lots of them. It tends to destroy or flush out or use up the B vitamins as well as magnesium, zinc and chromium. All of these nutrients, as we have seen, tend to aid blood pressure regulation.

Finally, and perhaps most importantly, sugar appears to have the same effect as salt, that is, it causes the tissues to retain water and in so doing to constrict. Experiments by biochemists at the University of Maryland and Michigan State University support this finding.

R. What evidence do you have regarding sugar's effect on humans?

A. Quite a bit. We do know that people who eat a good deal of sugar suffer many more heart attacks and the discrepancy between them and low sugar eaters in this respect cannot be fully explained by their greater tendency to be overweight. A British physician named John Yudkin has done extensive and intensive research on this point. Dr. Yudkin and his co-workers have found that a person consuming four ounces of sugar a day has five times as much chance of developing a heart attack as a person whose sugar consumption is only two ounces a day.

R. How much sugar does the average American consume?

A. More than four ounces a day. Dr. Yudkin has also turned up all kinds of other data to underscore his point. For example, he and his associates examined the sugar eating habits of two groups of patients at a London hospital. The first group were admitted for heart and arterial problems; the second group were admitted for accidents. The first group of patients ate, on the average, twice as much sugar as the accident victims. What's more, a closer look at the sugar eaters showed that in each and every one "the degree of atherosclerosis was proportional to the amount of dietary sugar." To put it more simply, those among them who ate more sugar had greater heart and arterial problems than those who ate less.

Finally, Yudkin and many others as well have observed that throughout the world, the heart attack rate seems to correlate much more strongly with sugar consumption than it does with fat consumption. Yemenite Jews, for example, when they migrate to Israel, start to eat much more refined sugar while their fat consumption, if anything, tends to go down. Yet their heart attack rate goes up markedly.

R. I notice you keep mentioning "refined" sugar. What about brown sugar, corn syrup, maple syrup, molasses and honey? Do these sweeteners cause similar harm?

A. Corn syrup seems to be as injurious as refined sugar. Maple syrup is somewhat better since it comes wrapped up with the various nutrients present in the syrup itself. Brown sugar is not raw sugar but simply white sugar that has been coated with molasses. Molasses is a food which is rich in many minerals such as iron and calcium. It also contains good quantities of the B vitamins. It can be considered, on the whole, as a fairly healthful food. Its use in producing brown sugar, however, is not sufficient to make brown sugar a healthful food, though it does reduce to some degree the harmfulness of the original refined sugar. As noted in Chapter 3, Dr. Schroeder found that brown sugar that had been so heavily coated with molasses that it would tend to stick together did not deplete the body of chromium. White sugar, as you may recall, does have this undesirable effect.

As to honey's action on the human system, this remains something of a mystery. We do know that most, though certainly not all, of the sugar in honey is what is called a simple sugar. This means that unlike refined sugar or the sugar in molasses or maple syrup, it does not require the elaborate conversion process. To put it differently, much of the sugars in honey can pass directly into the system without the pancreas having to pump out much insulin. Also, honey comes wrapped up with various nutrients, not all of which have been analyzed. Many feel that these properties make it more acceptable to the body. Some even go so far as to claim that honey produces positive benefits. There is some evidence that beekeepers tend to live to advanced ages and that they enjoy an amazingly low cancer rate. For example, a French study of the deaths of 1,000 beekeepers found that only one of them had died of cancer. But whether these beneficial phenomena result from eating honey remains to be seen.

R. I would suppose that you would not approve of saccharin since so much evidence has arisen as to its tendency to cause cancer?

A. The evidence is not completely convincing. It is true that feeding animals saccharin-saturated diets has succeeded in raising their rates of bladder cancer. But no evidence has turned up to show that human saccharin-users have higher rates of bladder cancer than those who don't use this sweetener. The latest study, published in the *Journal of the American Medical Association* in mid 1978, concluded that saccharin was not likely to be cancer-causing in man, at least at the levels at which it is customarily consumed. Sugar, on the other hand, has been heavily implicated in cancer. Three separate studies have shown that sugar weakens the human immunization system and the proper functioning of this system is believed crucial to cancer control. Furthermore, a study by the British Cancer Institute found sugar to be the foremost dietary cause of breast cancer. (Fat placed second on the dietary causation list for this illness.)

When one takes into account these factors along with sugar's detrimental effect on the heart, arteries and blood pressure mechanism, it would appear to be far more lethal than saccharin. This is not to say in the slightest that saccharin is good for you. Far from it. But compared to sugar, its effects seem almost benign. One further thing about saccharin. There is evidence that vitamin C taken in substantial amounts dislodges any amount of saccharin that may accumulate in the bladder. So if you are getting your vitamin C in the amounts recommended in Chapter 4, you are acquiring some protection against any negative consequences which the artificial sweetener may create.

R. Why do the authorities make such a fuss about saccharin and say little or nothing about sugar?

A. One reason is that there is specific legislation requiring them to proscribe any manufactured food that has in any way been found to contain any substance which can be termed carcinogenic or cancer-causing. Not being a manufactured food, even though it is a highly processed one, sugar does not fall within that framework. Furthermore, most doctors as we have sadly seen, know little and care less about nutrition, with the result that only a small number have familiarized themselves with the vast body of research regarding the harmful effects of sugar. Some pediatricians even reward their young patients with lollipops. Finally, and perhaps most importantly, the sugar lobby is one of the most powerful interest groups in Washington. It may sound unbelievable but we American consumers/taxpayers now pay out through subsidies and above-market prices nearly a half billion dollars a year to protect sugar farmers and processors.

R. What about meat? I'm not talking now about the salted or processed meats which you earlier identified as harmful, nor about the organ meats such as liver and kidneys which you pinpointed as being helpful, in blood pressure control. I mean the roasts, steaks and chops which the average American commonly eats, at least when he or she can afford them. Do these kinds of meats boost blood pressure?

A. There's a good deal of dispute and debate on this question. Studies going back to the 1920s have consistently shown vegetarians to have lower blood pressures than meat eaters. This has obviously impressed upon many the notion that meat generally elevates blood pressure. What has made the case against meat even more persuasive is that some of these studies seem to have succeeded in factoring out some of the other factors which could influence the problem. By that I mean that they have allowed for such factors as the differences between vegetarians and non-vegetarians in such areas as smoking, drinking and good health habits generally. Even when such differences are taken into account, the vegetarians have come out on top.

For example, a study which appeared in the March, 1978 issue of *Preventive Medicine* compared 86 Mormons with 86 Seventh-Day Adventists. Both groups follow essentially similar life styles with no smoking, no drinking and so forth. The only difference is that Seventh-Day Adventists do not generally eat meat while Mormons do. The investigation showed that the vegetarian Adventists enjoyed significantly lower blood pressures than the meat-eating Mormons. The Adventists also had lower cholesterol levels and lower cancer rates.

Another study conducted by a team of Harvard Medical School researchers a few years earlier focused on a group of young people, many of whom were vegetarians. The researchers weighed all the factors they could think of that could influence blood pressure such as smoking, salt, sugar, etc. Their findings?

Meat, in and of itself, not only caused blood pressure to rise but it seemed to do so more than the other factors they had allowed for. To put it differently, meat correlated more closely with HBP than smoking, salt, sugar, etc. This study was reported in the *American Journal of Epidemiology* of November, 1974.

R. Such studies would seem to clinch the case against meat.

A. Not quite. As I said earlier the question remains a highly controversial one. Eskimos living in inland areas, for example, eat huge quantities of meat but show no signs of higher blood pressure. Dr. Robert Atkins of New York City has put thousands of people on high-protein diets on which they eat lots of meat. Yet he insists that he has found no evidence whatsoever that such diets elevated their blood pressures. And many respected health writers claim that any linkage thought to exist between meat and high blood pressure is based on a misreading of the facts.

One of these writers, Ruth Adams, points out that vegetarians ingest a lot of fiber and this may have made the difference in such studies as I just cited. Eskimos and other primitive or traditional peoples consume a lot of fiber in their meat for they eat the bones, gristle and even some fur and feathers. Thus, it may be the fiberless form in which meat is marketed today that spells the difference.

R. What, then, do you suggest?

A. I would imagine that one could eat moderate amounts of most meats without undue danger. But I would favor the low-fat meats such as turkey, chicken and lamb as well as the organ meats previously cited. And of course one should stay clear of the processed and/or heavily salted meats that were mentioned earlier.

R. What about preservatives? You mentioned them as another enemy in the blood pressure battle. Are all of them harmful?

A. When it comes to HBP, it's the nitrites and nitrates that do the most harm. These substances seem injurious in themselves but their detrimental effect is increased by the fact that they are customarily compounded with sodium. Indeed, any preservative with sodium in its name should be consumed in only minute amounts, if at all.

R. What about other preservatives?

A. There is some evidence that many of them may raise blood pressure. A California allergist named Ben Feingold some years ago reported finding that hyperactive children often became much calmer when additives, especially certain coloring agents, were removed from their food. A Connecticut physician, Dr. James A. Harkins, claims to have achieved surprising success in lowering blood pressure by the same means. He says his high blood pressure and heart patients even undergo personality changes when placed on a additive-free diet. They become far less nervous and tense. They also suffer far fewer heart attacks. In an interview with *Prevention* (June 1978), he said "I used to have about six (heart attacks) a year among my patients. But since I started using this diet, about four years ago, there has been only one. Not one per year, but one, *total*, during the whole four years. That's quite a reduction." (emphasis in the original)

Obviously the whole subject needs further study. But the evidence available so far indicates that we should keep our intake of additives to a minimum.

R. I find it interesting that it was an allergist who first noticed a possible connection between food additives and hyperactive behavior. Isn't that a bit unusual?

A. Not at all. And that conveniently brings us to the next topic for consideration, namely food allergies and HBP.

R. You mean hay fever has a relationship to blood pressure?

A. Allergies cover many more medical phenomena than hay fever. Many people are allergic to various foods and their reaction can take the form of an elevated blood pressure. One hypertension specialist reports seeing a patient's systolic pressure shoot up from normal to 230 about six hours after eating wheat.

R. But several times earlier in our discussions you cited wheat, at least the unprocessed kind, as helpful to high blood pressure. Now you say it raises blood pressure.

A. It did so in this particular patient who happened to be allergic to it. Some people are even allergic to certain fillers in vitamins. Don't forget that every single person is biochemically unique.

R. How can I tell if I am allergic to certain foods and, if so, what foods?

A. There is a simple, though somewhat controversial, test that you can administer to yourself. It was developed by Dr. Arthur F. Coca, a former honorary president of the American Association of Immunology. If you suspect that certain foods are causing you problems, then limit your meals for a day to those foods. Take your pulse on arising and then again just before your first meal. After eating one of the suspected foods take your pulse twice, first right after the meal and then again an hour later. Do the same with the other foods as you proceed throughout the day. Any foods you are allergic to will cause your pulse rate to increase.

Further details can be found in Dr. Coca's interesting book *The Pulse Test*. However, I should point out that the test does not work for everyone. Some people experience higher pulse rates after every meal regardless of what they eat.

R. But I thought we were concerned with blood pressure, not pulse rate.

A. They are, to be sure, different but they are hardly unrelated. A high pulse rate is quite common among those with high blood pressure and steps taken to lower one will frequently lower the other. Dr. Coca makes this point in his book. So if a particular food is stepping up your pulse rate it is probably causing other harmful effects as well, including higher blood pressure.

R. So far you have said nothing about such things as coffee or alcohol. I should think that for a person concerned with keeping his blood pressure down, coffee and alcohol would really be bad news.

A. The news about these two controversial foods is not so bad as you may think. In 1978 two reassuring studies came to light concerning coffee. One was a survey of over 2,500 people, Blacks and Whites, in Evans County, Georgia. It found no consistent differences in the deaths from heart disease between heavy coffee drinkers and those who drank less or none at all. The other study consisted of more than 72,000 employees at IBM. This investigation showed that the blood pressure readings, both systolic and diastolic, of those who drank a good deal of coffee averaged about the same as those who drank little or no coffee. This study appeared in the *New England Journal of Medicine*.

R. You mean I can drink all the coffee I want without having to worry about ill effects?

A. No. Coffee does appear to have other undesirable consequences even if it does not raise blood pressure. It may tend to destroy or drive out B vitamins from the body and to increase blood sugar. Some research suggests, but does not prove, that coffee may be implicated in bladder cancer and prostate problems. And don't forget that coffee stimulates the system not by adding any nourishment but, in a sense, by flogging it. Finally, it is at least mildly addictive. However, if a person really insists on drinking coffee, he or she can probably consume one or two or possibly three cups a day without doing themselves any great damage providing the other factors in their diets are good.

R. What about alcohol?

A. Here the news, or at least some of the news, is actually positive. In the early 1970s, doctors at the Kaiser-Permanente Medical Center in California found that an unusually high number of their heart attack patients were teetotlers. This prompted them to look further. They reviewed the medical records of 120,000 patients and found that moderate drinkers experienced 30 per cent *fewer* heart attacks than non-drinkers. The moderate drinkers had lower blood pressures as well.

R. What about the not-so-moderate drinkers?

Q. Theirs was a different story. They fared worse than the non-drinkers. The cut-off point seemed to be two drinks a day. Anyone downing three or more drinks a day was likely to have higher blood pressure and a higher likelihood of a heart attack.

R. What about other studies? Do they confirm these findings?

A. They most assuredly do. Researchers at the Medical College of Wisconsin, for example, measured the blockage in the coronary arteries of moderate drinkers compared to total abstainers. They found that the drinkers had the healthier arteries. And a study of 7,705 Japanese men in Hawaii found that those who drank three bottles of beer a day had half as much coronary heart disease and only one-fifth the heart attack rate as those who drank no alcohol at all.

R. Does this mean that beer is the best thing to drink?

A. Not necessarily. Wine, especially red wine, may offer the most benefits. Wine, as you know, comes from grapes and grapes, as we saw earlier, contain a great deal of potassium and almost no sodium. Then, in 1977, *Science News* reported a Canadian study which found that grapes contain certain compounds which have an anti-viral activity. In other words, they act as virus killers. And wine itself seems to have a beneficial effect on the digestive process. Wasn't it Saint Paul who said "Drink a little wine for thy stomach's sake?"

It is interesting to note in this connection that in the region in Southern Russia where so many people live to such advanced ages, alcohol made from grapes is a staple in the diet. Not only is wine consumed with lunch and dinner but a small amount of vodka is also drunk, and this vodka comes from grapes.

R. You indicated that red wine may be better than white. Why?

A. The Canadian study found that red wines have stronger anti-viral activity. Also such wines contain greater amounts of iron and other vital minerals. But both kinds of wine and alcohol generally, when consumed with caution, may lead to greater health and happiness. As you can see, a longer life doesn't have to be an unpleasant one.

CHAPTER 6

Myths of the Heart: Fats, Eggs and Exercise

R. First what do you mean by "Myths of the Heart?"

A. Simply that there are many ideas being spread around by doctors and others regarding heart health that are simply not true. One of the most fashionable and dangerous of these notions is that polyunsaturated or vegetable fats are much better for you than saturated or animal fats. The evidence clearly demonstrates that this is not necessarily so. Indeed, the reverse may be true.

R. I have certainly heard of this "myth," as you call it. But this so-called myth is supported by the American Heart Association and some of the country's leading cardiologists. So why do you call it a myth?

A. Studies have been made of Eskimos, men of the

Maseai tribes in Kenya and Tanzania and of immigrant Italians in the United States. All of these groups consume diets high in saturated fats; all of them suffer fewer heart problems than other groups with lower intakes of saturated fats.

In India, an even sharper discrepancy between saturated fat consumption and heart illness has been found. The Punjabis who live in northern India and northeastern Pakistan eat a lot of saturated fat. Unsaturated fat, on the other hand, makes up no more than 2 per cent of their diet. In southern India, however, there is a group called the Gujaratis who pursue a diametrically opposite dietary pattern. Unsaturated fats constitute 44 per cent of their food intake. Yet the Gujaratis, with more than 20 times the unsaturated fat consumption of the Punjabis, *suffer 15 times as much heart disease*.

Then there is a group of Polynesians who live principally on coconuts. Now, the coconut is the one plant food which is high in saturated fat and thus saturated fat is believed to make up almost 80 per cent of the diet of this Polynesian group. Yet, they have been found to have the lowest pulse rate and lowest cholesterol of any group ever studied.

Finally, I should like to call attention to the fact that in World War II, the margarine plants in Norway were destroyed while those in England continued to operate. The result: the incidence of arterial disease went down in Norway while it rose in England.

R. But surely there is evidence to support the current, wide-spread belief that vegetable fats are beneficial to the heart?

A. Yes, but on closer examination this evidence has been found to be grievously flawed.

Perhaps the study most often cited to support this theory about the desirability of vegetable fats was a research project undertaken at a Los Angeles veterans hospital in the late 1960s. Nearly 1,000 veterans were divided into two groups. One group was put on a diet high in vegetable fats while the second group was allowed to eat what was called the standard American diet. At the end of a five-year period, it was found that the vegetable oil eaters had experienced substantially fewer fatal heart attacks.

R. Well, if in matching two groups of men, we find that those eating a diet high in vegetable oils suffer substantially fewer heart attacks, then, so it would seem to me, we have proven a valuable point.

A. So it also seemed to the two doctors who conducted the study. But some follow-up investigation has shown that the two groups were not evenly matched. The group that continued to eat the customary American diet, so it has been found, contained a great many more heavy cigarette smokers than did the vegetable oil eaters. It also contained almost double the number of veterans over 80 years of age. Once allowance was made for these factors, no difference in the heart disease death rate was discerned. Regrettably, the results of this subsequent investigation have received much less attention and are much less well known than the initial, faulty findings.

R. What about other studies?

A. There are two or three other ones which, viewed superficially, seemed to support the unsaturated fat thesis. But these have also been shown to contain fatal flaws.

R. But haven't the number of fatal heart attacks in the U.S. gone down overall in recent years? And hasn't the consumption of unsaturated fats increased at the same time? This would seem to present fairly convincing proof of the protection which such fats provide.

A. From 1910 to about 1970, the amount of polyunsaturated fats in the American diet just about doubled. This growth pattern was accompanied by an equally impressive growth in the incidence of heart disease. In the 1970s, some fall-off in the fatal heart attack rate began to be noticed. But when one considers how many Americans, especially middle-age males, had by then given up cigarette smoking, one can only wonder why the drop wasn't greater. And don't forget that the 1970s witnessed a startling surge of interest in health and health foods. Millions of Americans, for instance, are now taking vitamins and minerals that, as we saw earlier, help protect the heart.

R. Still, I find it hard to believe that the American Heart Association and most cardiologists would go on urging us to eat more vegetable fats if the evidence really points in the other direction.

A. Your qualms on this point are quite understandable. But don't forget that the Heart Association takes its cues from the cardiologists. And as for the cardiologists, they, like most doctors, indeed like most people, find it excruciatingly difficult to change long standing beliefs.

R. But if the facts are as you say they are, then surely some voices would have been raised in the medical world against the prevailing notions about polyunsaturates.

A. Some voices have been raised. Dr. Roger Williams, the highly esteemed biochemist whom I cited earlier, feels that the evidence indicates that consumption of large amounts of vegetable oils place those who consume them in greater peril. He maintains that "individuals who ingest a large amount of polyunsaturated fats on the notion that it will protect them against atherosclerosis and coronary heart disease may actually be exposing themselves to the disease"!

R. Dr. Williams may be an eminent biochemist but he is not a physician. Have any medical doctors, especially cardiologists, taken a similar stand?

A. They certainly have. One of them is Dr. Mark D. Altschule, a cardiologist who is on the faculty of both the Harvard and Yale Medical Schools. Dr. Altschule may be the only cardiologist in the country who has focused his attention almost exclusively on the role of nutritional factors in heart health. Thus, he probably can lay claim to greater qualifications to speak out on this point than any one else. And Dr. Altschule has published a good deal of well-documented work designed to prove the fallacy of popular notions regarding oils and the heart. To him these notions represent superstition, not science.

Dr. George V. Mann, the research physician who was cited in an earlier chapter concerning his work with yogurt and cholesterol also takes issue with the belief in unsaturates. He refers to it as a "dietary dogma" which, he says, has been a "money-maker for segments of the food industry" and a "fund-raiser for the American Heart Association." Dr. Mann's remarks were made at a symposium sponsored by the Boston University School of Medicine in the summer of 1978. According to newspaper accounts of the conclave, most of the other panelists agreed with him.

R. If the case against the vegetable fats is as strong as you claim, then how did the belief in their desirability arise in the first place?

A. Early experiments showed that consumption of unsaturated fats could lower the cholesterol deposits in the blood. The reductions were modest, ranging, usually, up to 15 per cent in those whose cholesterol was high to begin with and who would then consume such fats in heavy amounts. Still, such a reduction would take place.

Now, cholesterol is a fat-like substance which can lodge on the walls of the arteries, narrowing the passageways and causing possible damage to the arterial wall. People with high amounts of cholesterol in their blood do show somewhat greater susceptibility to heart attacks. Consequently, anything that could help clear the blood of excessive cholesterol was considered beneficial in preventing atherosclerosis and heart ailments. Unfortunately, it hasn't worked out that way.

R. Any idea why it hasn't?

A. Ideas, yes, but a firm, fact-based explanation, no. There is some evidence, so far only slight, that suggests that the unsaturated fats may reduce cholesterol in the blood only by actually depositing it on the arterial walls. But I wish to emphasize that this theory remains only slightly supported as yet.

What we have found out is that the whole subject of cholesterol is far more controversial and complex than was originally thought. While there is a statistical relationship between high blood cholesterol and heart disease it is not by any means a perfect one. Most heart attack victims have normal cholesterol levels and some people with high cholesterol levels enjoy normal blood pressure and long lives free of heart problems. There is also evidence that only certain forms of cholesterol endanger the arteries and heart while other forms actually seem to be beneficial. In any case, the presence of large amounts of cholesterol in the bloodstream, even if it is of the detrimental form, should not be viewed as actually causing atherosclerosis. Rather, its presence is a symptom of something else that is wrong, and reducing or raising the blood cholesterol itself will not greatly affect the more basic problem which is producing it. You may want to think of cholesterol in this sense as a barometer. We know that a falling barometer will presage a storm, but we also know that pushing down the barometer needle will not, in itself, produce a storm and pushing it up won't prevent one.

R. Do you mean that we can eat all the saturated fat we want without fear of the consequences?

A. No. Although some groups seem to be able to eat a lot of saturated fat with relative impunity, nevertheless a high consumption of either saturated or in certain forms, unsaturated fat can cause or contribute to many health disorders, including cancer. We shall be taking a closer look at this problem in the last chapter.

At present fat of all kinds makes up over 40 per cent

of the calories in the average American's daily diet. We would do well to reduce its share to 20 per cent. This represents the average level of fat intake in Japan, and the Japanese, despite a lot of salt-induced high blood pressure, and despite their highly polluted environment, enjoy a much longer life span than we do.

R. Are there any particular fats that are better than others for us to eat?

A. Probably the best is butterfat. It aids and abets the absorption of calcium, increases the growth of certain favorable bacteria in the intestine—don't forget that some bacteria are beneficial to human health—and helps the system synthesize certain B vitamins, especially B6. Butterfat also contains some valuable trace elements. Laboratory animals fed a diet supplemented with butterfat-containing whole milk grow faster and seem more robust than those whose diet has been supplemented with only skim milk. After surveying all the evidence, including the evidence presented earlier comparing heart attack rates among various groups, Dr. Williams goes so far to say that "Butterfat, itself, appears to protect *against* atherosclerosis."

R. I suppose from what you have said that we should avoid unsaturated fats like the plague.

A. No. They provide certain nutritious acids which the human system needs. What we should try to avoid are what are called hydrogenated fats. The hydrogenation process enables fats to stay on the store shelf longer without turning rancid. However, it also makes these fats much more harmful. The way it does this is too complex for us to go into but that it does do this is attested to by Dr. Altschule and many other researchers. Margarine, to take a prime example of a hydrogenated fat, *increases* atherosclerosis in laboratory animals. Margarine represents one unsaturated fat product that should be avoided like the plague.

R. Let's pass on to the second subject you list under myths of the heart, namely eggs. Now eggs, so I understand, contain not just fat but cholesterol itself. Are you going to say that eggs, like saturated fats, do not necessarily harm the heart?

A. I plan to go farther than that and claim that eggs, on the whole, tend to protect the heart.

To begin with, eggs, though they contain cholesterol, do not appreciably increase blood cholesterol in the average human being. Researchers at Mt. Sinai Hospital in New York first discovered this in 1953. They found that feeding eggs to volunteer subjects would cause a sudden elevation in their cholesterol count but that the effect was only temporary. Within a few hours the cholesterol level would fall back to where it was before the eggs were consumed.

Since then a flock of studies have appeared showing essentially the same thing. To take just one of them, four research physicians at the University of Michigan did an extensive dietary survey of the residents of a whole community (Tecumseh, Michigan). Among other things, they found no relationship between the amount of cholesterol in the diet and the amount of cholesterol in the blood. Those who ate a lot of cholesterol-rich foods such as eggs or liver did not, on the average, have higher cholesterol levels than those who ate less of or even avoided such foods. The results of this survey were published, by the way, in the *Journal of the American*

Medical Association on October 25, 1976.

R. Why, then, hasn't the medical profession changed its position on eggs?

A. As I noted earlier, none of us find it easy to give up long and deeply held beliefs. For the medical profession, it would be doubly difficult for it would have to concede that it had been giving the American public bad medical advice all along. The same problem has doubtlessly prevented it from accepting the fact that their advice on unsaturated fats has also been wrong.

R. However, you quoted some authorities, rather good ones, as accepting, as you put it, the "facts" about unsaturated fats. Do they also accept these "facts" regarding the harmlessness of eggs?

A. Yes. In a book entitled *Nutritional Factors in General Medicine* and written for his fellow physicians, Dr. Mark D. Altschule observes "one of the ideas current in this country is that eating cholesterol (or other substances that are said to interact with cholesterol such as saturated fats) cause the atherosclerosis responsible for heart attacks, strokes and so forth. The notion has no substantial backing; that is whatever data have been brought forward to support it are found, on examination, either not to support it *or to contradict it.*" (My emphasis).

R. That last phrase, "contradict it", intrigues me. It would seem to imply that the data not only absolves eggs from the charge of causing atherosclerosis but indicates that they may even help prevent it.

110

A. You infer correctly. The evidence strongly suggests that eggs, far from hurting the heart, actually help it. Let me cite just two examples.

A physician named Sam Berman once put 400 overweight and middle-aged Boston policemen on a weight-reducing diet. As part of the diet they were instructed to eat several eggs a day. At the end of eight years none of these 400 middle-aged men, all of whom were in a stressful occupation, had had a heart attack.

A still more startling discovery was made by two physicians who were carrying out a survey for the American Cancer Society. They checked the dietary intake against the medical records of 800,409 people over a six-year period. They found, among other things, that those who ate five or more eggs a week suffered fewer, far fewer, heart attacks than those who consumed less than five eggs a week.

R. How do you explain such remarkable results?

A. When we were discussing the beneficial effects of lecithin, I pointed out that eggs were the richest source of this fat-emulsifying nutrient. It undoubtedly contributes to the effectiveness of eggs in helping the heart. Then, eggs contain a lot of trace minerals. These include such useful ones as selenium and zinc that we examined earlier. It also includes one we did not discuss, namely silicon. Not too much is known about silicon and its relationship to health but one interesting and possibly important fact has come to light: Atherosclerotic blood vessels show signs of severe silicon depletion. There may also be other factors involved that we don't know about. What we do know is that the best evidence tends to give eggs a clean bill of health as far as human health is concerned.

R. But, surely those medical people who are constantly urging us to cut down on eggs are not proceeding on pure theory alone. Don't they have evidence they can cite to back up their claims?

A. Remarkably little. And such evidence as they do have comes mostly from dubious animal experiments. Researchers have found that feeding certain animals huge amounts of cholesterol will increase the level of cholesterol in their blood. But the amounts given are often what would represent the equivalent of 40 eggs a day for a human adult. Furthermore, these animals are usually vegetarians who cannot metabolize eggs. But most importantly the cholesterol utilized in these experiments is not in the same form as that found in eggs. It has been exposed to the air, often for long periods of time, and this causes it to change in undesirable ways.

Dr. Altschule has called attention to this commonly overlooked fact. He draws from it the lesson that eggs, too, under certain conditions may cause cholesterol to rise. This may occur when they are consumed in the form of dried egg yolks such as are found in many pastries. *In this form*, he says, eggs could prove harmful. Otherwise, he, along with others who have seriously investigated the question, see no ill effects for the average person through the eating of eggs.

The health magazine *Today's Living* once reported the case of a 63-year-old Australian who, because of certain throat problems, could eat nothing but raw eggs. He was therefore downing about 72 eggs a week. Yet, he seemed to be not only surviving but even thriving on this regimen.

R. You have made a pretty good case against un-

saturated fats and for eggs but I think that with this next "myth" you are attempting to expose, you are going to have problems. If there is one thing that almost all authorities are agreed upon, it is the value of exercise.

A. Allow me to qualify your statement. What almost all authorities agree upon is the value of physical activity. I couldn't agree more myself. But physical activity is not the same thing as exercise, especially when the exercise takes the vigorous, competitive form that it so often takes today.

R. But isn't there a lot of evidence to back up the exercise enthusiasts?

A. Actually, there is surprisingly little. Most of the studies cited to support the claims for exercise deal only with physical activity. For example, the AMA likes to call attention to a study of San Francisco longshoremen which showed that those whose jobs required heavy physical work suffered far fewer heart attacks than those whose jobs were less demanding. I have no fault to find with this research. But I question whether its findings can be interpreted as bolstering the value of vigorous exercise.

R. But haven't there been studies done on the effects of exercise itself?

A. There have been but these at best are inconclusive. Indeed, correctly interpreted they would seem to create suspicion rather than support.

For example, one study which was cited to me as a vindication of exercise compared the heart attack rates of men who exercised with those who didn't. The college professor who referred to this study said that it demonstrated that, while the exercisers suffered as many heart attacks as the non-exercisers, the attacks, on the whole, caused less damage to their hearts. I have never seen the study myself but, assuming it is true, then it would seem to show that exercise causes more harm than good.

R. Why do you say that?

A. When you compare two groups, you must take into account *all* the factors that may make them different. Now, a sample group of men who exercise is virtually certain to have fewer smokers, fewer heavy drinkers and fewer overweight members than a sample group of non-exercising men. Those who exercise on the average take greater care of their health in other ways than those who don't. Consequently, the fact that their heart attacks caused somewhat less damage should not be surprising. What should be surprising and even dismaying to exercise buffs is that their heart attack rate was no different than that of the non-exercisers. In view of their better health habits generally, it should be substantially lower. One could conclude from this study that exercise was actually causing heart attacks.

R. But surely there is no real evidence that exercise is bad for you.

A. Perhaps not. But there are plenty of indications that this could be the case, at least for many people. Another study tracked the medical history of 38,000 male college graduates. It revealed that those who played sports in college lived no longer than those who did not engage in athletics at all. Again we must take into account the differences between the groups. The athletes were probably healthier, as a group, to begin with. Those who were weak or sickly would probably be found in the non-athletic group. Furthermore, college athletes usually must follow rigid regimens that forbid smoking, drinking and late hours. Although many of them may take up these habits in later life, still the more dissolute and dissipated students would be likely to be found in the non-athletic group. Yet, despite their greater numbers of weak and sickly as well as dissolute and dissipated members, the non-athletic group equaled the athletic group in average life expectancy. This is hardly a vindication of the virtues of exercise.

No study that I know of has ever been made of professional athletes but such evidence as we have indicates, if anything, that their life spans fall below average. Only rarely do we find a professional athlete living into his 80s and almost never do we come across one who has survived until 90. Within a recent 20-month period, former Olympic Gold Medalist Ralph Metcalf, known as "the fastest human alive" died at 68; Gil Dodds, the clean-living minister who once held the world's record for the indoor mile run, died at age 58; and Neil Johnston, who won the National Basketball Association's scoring title three years, is now dead at age 49. All three were victims of heart attacks.

R. I notice that two of the three were runners. Does this mean that the current craze for jogging is dangerous?

A. Yes. Again, our evidence is not of the best but such as it is, it is scarcely reassuring. In Washington, D.C. during one week in October 1978, three middle-aged men, one of them a Congressman, dropped dead while jogging. All of them were seasoned joggers and the Congressman, Goodloe Byron of Maryland, had run in several marathons. Yet, he collapsed from a heart attack at the age of 49. The previous year, in a marathon in Hawaii, 100 out of the 3,000 contestants suffered heart attacks or other heart/circulatory problems before the race was over.

I remember reading somewhere that the middle-aged doctor who launched the whole jogging fad had also suffered a heart attack. From his hospital bed he was quoted as saying that he was going to reexamine his position on the subject.

R. But a lot of people do seem able to jog and engage in other vigorous sports into their 70s and 80s.

A. Yes, a lot of people can but apparently a lot can not. And those who can not seem to be much more numerous than most doctors have suspected.

R. Still, if vigorous exercise can prove so perilous to so many, as you contend, then surely some doctors must have observed it.

A. Some indeed have. One of these is San Francisco cardiologist Ray H. Rosenman. Dr. Rosenman has called jogging "a miserable post-collegiate athletic travesty." He contends that it has quite possibly killed hundreds of people.

R. If vigorous exercise can be as dangerous as you depict it to be, than what causes it to be so?

A. A Philadelphia physician named Hasib Tanyol

offers us a valuable clue. Dr. Tanyol, who has been a Professor of Medicine at two medical schools, once studied 298 college and professional football players. *He found that 26 per cent of them suffered from high blood pressure.* This is nearly *eight times* the incidence of HBP found in their age group. He also surveyed 60 college track-and-field athletes. Only 6.6 per cent of them had high blood pressure but even this was more than twice as high as the normal amount found in their age group.

R. Did Dr. Tanyol have an explanation for this?

A. He maintained that the increased incidence of high blood pressure resulted from the increased muscle which athletic activity builds. After all, muscle, like fat, needs to be nourished by the blood. Therefore, it can force the heart to pump harder.

Dr. William Weidman of the world-famed Mayo Clinic agrees with Dr. Tanyol, saying that his own research supports such a thesis. But I am not completely convinced that increased muscle is the sole explanation. Track athletes may have extra muscle but, at the same time, they also have less fat. In general they are thinner than most men their age. Consequently, if they have more than double the amount of high blood pressure for their age group, then other factors may also be at work.

R. What are these other factors?

A. Strenuous athletics, as you know, causes a lot of sweating. The body can lose a lot of valuable minerals in the lost perspiration. Among these lost minerals are potassium and magnesium. We have already seen how vital a role these two minerals play in regulating blood pressure.

R. But in perspiring doesn't the body lose sodium as well? Isn't this why athletes frequently take salt tablets?

A. Sodium does ooze out along with the potassium and magnesium in perspiration. But a study published in *Physiology Review* in 1978 demonstrated that relatively more fluid is lost than salt. The result is that the salt that remains in the systems becomes more concentrated and therefore more harmful.

R. So the loss of potassium and magnesium, accompanied by an increasing concentration of sodium, is one of the possible factors behind the higher incidence of HBP in athletes. What are the other factors?

A. There is only one other but this could be the most important of all.

Most athletic activity is intensely competitive. This includes even jogging for joggers are continually trying to increase their distance if not their speed. In one way or another they are often pushing themselves, in effect competing against themselves. The result of all this frantic and frequently frustrating effort is a lot of stress, and stress, as virtually every doctor will tell you, is a prime promoter of high blood pressure.

An interesting experiment along these lines was carried out by Dr. Gary Schwartz, a cardiologist at the Yale Medical School. He took a group of professional actors and asked them to think angry thoughts while exercising. He found that the exercise, coupled with the upsetting emotions, sent their blood pressure skyrocketing. He concluded that exercise was definitely doing them more harm than good.

R. I can imagine that the person playing golf or tennis, for example, does his blood pressure no good when he misses a shot.

A. This would seem to be likely. As a matter of fact, just tensing up to swing at the ball probably sends his blood pressure shooting up.

R. You did say earlier, however, that physical activity has been shown to be helpful to the heart and to health in general.

A. It most assuredly has. A 1974 Gallup poll of people 95 years of age and over found that continuous physical activity was the single greatest common denominator in their life style.

R. What kinds of physical activity seem best?

A. One of the very best seems to be the cheapest and easiest exercise of all, walking. *Executive Health*, a publication that probably boasts of the most impressive editorial board of any health publication in the world— it includes three Nobel prize winners in medicine—devoted its July, 1978 issure to celebrating the benefits of walking. Here is what it said. "Not running, not jogging, but *walking* is your most *efficient* form of exercise and the *only* one you can *safely* follow all the years of your life"! The emphasis on the words *walking*, *efficient*, etc. is theirs, not mine. It called walking, "Nature's own amazing anti-age antibiotic."

The case for walking rests on more than just theory,

expert opinion or anecdotal evidence. We have a very simple but very convincing statistic to back it up. This is the fact that the longest-lived occupational group in the United States are letter carriers. (Doctors, by the way, do not place anywhere near the top of the longevity list.)

There are many other forms of exercise which also seem to provide genuine health benefits to nearly all who practice them. Two examples are swimming and cross-country skiing. These rhythmic and generally non-competitive sports do not usually entail excessive mineral loss and excessive strain. In Roanoke, Virginia there is a woman who is still winning swimming meets at the age of 85, while in California, so I have heard, there is a man who is continuing to cross-country ski at the age of 103.

One final and all-too-often neglected form of physical activity also warrants support and that is dancing. It is certainly rhythmic and almost always non-competitive. To my knowledge no systematic study has ever been done concerning the death rates of dancers, but it is quite common to find professional dancers, unlike professional athletes, enjoying good health into their 80s and 90s. To take some examples from among movie stars, Fred Astaire and James Cagney are well past 80 while Bob Hope and Ray Bolger are in their late 70s. All of them seem to be enjoying remarkable health and vitality, with the possible exception of Mr. Cagney, who is diabetic. But at this writing even he is making a movie. The same goes for Gene Kelly, Ginger Rogers, Lucille Ball, Mickey Rooney, Donald O'Connor and many other professional dancers, all of whom are over 60.

One doesn't have to have any particular skill to enjoy the health benefits which dancing apparently bestows.

American Square dancing, for example, consists of a series of simple and largely mechanical steps. It is easily learned and easily done.

R. You would, however, warn people away from such sports as tennis, golf and jogging?

A. Not necessarily. But I would urge them to proceed with great caution. Any person, especially any older person, who pursues such sports should make sure that their mineral intake is more than adequate. More importantly, they should make sure that their attitude is reasonably relaxed. With the proper frame of mind, many of the dangers which competitive or strenuous sports pose can be substantially reduced. Nevertheless, these sports will probably remain less congenial to the human system than the others I have mentioned. In earlier chapters, we saw that the human body seems to respond more favorably to the more natural forms of food. It would appear that the same holds true for the more natural forms of exercise as well.

CHAPTER 7

Weight, Tobacco
and Stress

R. How important a factor is weight in blood pressure control?

A. Its importance would be difficult to exaggerate. Every extra pound of tissue, whether muscle or fat, needs an additional mile of blood vessels for its nourishment, and remember that the heart must pump blood through those additional blood vessels from 50 to 100 times a minute. Thus, the more we weigh, the more work our hearts must perform.

R. However, not every fat person suffers from high blood pressure and not every thin person can boast of low blood pressure.

A. True. Still a clear-cut correlation exists. From ages 20 to 40, the rate of hypertension found among overweight individuals is double that found among those of normal weight. From 40 to 60, the HBP rate is 50 per cent greater among the overweight.

Doctors have achieved some remarkable successes in reducing HBP simply by reducing weight. An Israeli medical team put a group of 24 overweight HBP patients on a reducing diet that caused most of them to lose 20 pounds. In nearly all cases, blood pressure levels fell to normal in those who lost this amount of weight. Another group of patients who were given drugs designed to lower HBP did not fare anywhere near as well. The doctor who headed the experiment concluded that "Weight control seems to offer an efficient, low-cost means of blood pressure control that is free of side effects and often makes it possible to avoid medication or to institute a lower dose of medication."

R. That's all well and good but aren't some people congenitally disposed toward being overweight? We all know people who eat a great deal and don't gain weight and other people who eat less but who always seem to be fighting the "battle of the bulge."

A. It is true that the metabolism of certain individuals allows them to burn up energy more easily than others. But the differences are frequently exaggerated. Overweight people usually eat more than others. And while fat people may have fat children, thus indicating a genetic disposition to obesity, they also, as Dr. Altschule has pointed out, tend to have fat pets. In other words, food habits not genetic inheritance generally determines whether we will weigh more than we should.

One inherent, inborn factor does play a significant role, however, and that is sex. Women tend to be naturally fatter than men and to have a harder time losing weight than do most men. Nature has given them an extra layer of fat to protect their unborn offspring once they become pregnant. This layer of fat, according to

Dr. Barbara Edelstein of Mt. Sinai Hospital in New York, remains in place whether or not they ever become pregnant. From 15 to 30 per cent of the average adult woman's body weight consists of fat. This compares to only 10 to 15 per cent for men.

This does not mean that a woman can not and should not lose weight if her poundage exceeds the amount her doctor deems desirable, nor does it mean that her mate can ignore his own problems in that department. Most American men, like most American women, are overweight. What's more, the situation concerning male obesity seems to be getting worse, not better. From 1968 to 1978, the average American male put on six additional and unnecessary pounds.

R. Several diets have been proposed in recent years for quick weight loss. Which of these diets is best?

A. One should be wary of all crash diets designed to shed weight quickly. Most of the pounds lost consist of the body's fluid and carbohydrate stores. These losses do not represent actual fat reduction. Furthermore, they are all too easily replenished once the diet is over.

These diets also frequently deprive the system of needed nutrients. Furthermore, they may lead to an even greater weight gain later on. Dr. Bela Szepesi, a scientist with the U.S. Department of Agriculture, told a conference in 1978 that restricted food intake appears to trigger a mechanism that will actually overstimulate the appetite once the diet is over. We know that about 95 per cent of all people who successfully subject themselves to crash diets eventually end up as heavy, if not more heavy, than they were before.

For those concerned with lowering their blood pressure, such sudden, all-out diets may prove particularly troublesome. The stress produced from swinging from one type of dietary situation to the other, may in itself raise the blood pressure. Experiments carried out with dogs and young swine show that repeated episodes of starvation and refeeding will elevate blood pressure considerably. Moreover, prisoners of war who have lived under conditions of semi-starvation show a distinct proneness to developing high blood pressure once they have become liberated and can eat all they want.

R. What, then, is the solution?

A. The solution is to set up a diet in which one can lose weight gradually. It should be a diet that one can more or less follow for life.

R. I have heard that protein foods should be the basis for a weight-controlling diet. Is that correct?

A. Whether high protein consumption has a beneficial or baneful effect on humans has not been determined. We do know that when protein consumption exceed 90 grams a day, the system starts to excrete certain valuable minerals. Such a high level of protein ingestion also increases the body's need for vitamin A. And some physicians feel that too much protein can place an undue stain on the kidneys.

We also know that in those two regions of the world where people are reputed to live the longest—the district in southern Russia mentioned earlier as well as the Hunza section of Pakistan—protein consumption tends to be on the low side. Of course, it should be noted that the people of Hunza do not have sufficient land in which to raise animals, so their meat-eating is confined mostly to celebrations. Also, back in June, 1968 *Nutrition To-*

day reported an experiment conducted by a Swedish physician in which a group of subjects showed reduced physical stamina after being placed on a high-protein, high-fat diet.

Nevertheless, the evidence remains far from conclusive. The Eskimos are probably the world's premier protein eaters and not only do they exhibit all the favorable health patterns I mentioned earlier but they also show no signs of lacking physical endurance. Far from it. And again, Dr. Atkins, along with some others who favor high protein diets, claims to have found no unfavorable results.

But whether high-protein diets offer any perils to our health or not, another and less controversial diet exists for helping us control our weight.

R. What is it?

A. The high-fiber diet, that is a diet consisting largely, or at least heavily, of fruits, vegetables and whole grains.

R. That sounds strange. Admittedly, you have already indicated that such foods can help lower blood pressure in other ways but I would not think their consumption would lead to weight loss. Fruits contain sugar while whole grains consist largely of carbohydrates. I would think that this would rule them out as weight-reducers.

A. The sugar in fruit consists largely of fructose, and fructose differs in some important ways from the sucrose which makes up ordinary table sugar. Fructose is absorbed into the bloodstream more slowly. It also is much sweeter, on a calorie-for-calorie basis, than sucrose. As a result, it dampens hunger pangs much more effectively. A piece of fruit such as a raw prune eaten before a meal can help us reach the satiety level sooner. I mean by this that it can help us reach the point of feeling filled up before we have eaten too much.

As for whole grains, they are, to be sure, carbohydrates. But that doesn't make them fattening. Experiments at the University of Michigan and at the University of Southern California show that student volunteers instructed to eat seven slices of whole grain bread a day will lose weight *regardless of what else they might eat*.

R. Are you trying to tell me that eating lots of bread can actually cause someone to lose weight?

A. Yes, especially when it is whole grain bread. The weight losses experienced on such diets were not spectacular. They averaged a little less than a pound a week. Yet, the loss did take place. Eating seven slices of whole grain bread a day will produce an average weight loss of seven pounds in two months.

Fibrous foods such as whole grains ter.d to help us keep down weight in two ways. First, they speed the transit of food through the system. This keeps a lot of the food from becoming absorbed. Secondly, and most importantly, they tend to give us a filled-up feeling so that we naturally eat less of any food. Try eating seven slices of whole grain bread a day and you'll see.

R. What about snacking between meals? Most doctors frown on this practice and say it leads to increased weight.

A. If you snack on candy or pastries or similar types of food, it certainly will. But if you eat wholesome snacks, then on the contrary, snacking will help you shed excess poundage. Indeed, if you are really serious about becoming and staying thin, then you would do well to eat more frequently, perhaps six small meals a day.

R. Why is that?

A. The body's capacity to burn off calories diminishes as the number of calories poured into it at any one time increases. This is especially true as we get older and our system's ability to process fat and other foods tends to decline. But even at younger ages, we do a better job in dissipating the calories we consume when we spread them out.

Many of the medical authorities cited earlier wholeheartedly agree on this point. Dr. Hrachovec observes that "an unusually high level of triglycerides (fats) and glucose (sugar) in the blood can cause a traffic jam: more fuel is being dumped into the blood stream than can be unloaded and used in tissue cells." The result, he says, is a stored-up surplus which we call fat.

Dr. Altschule shares these sentiments. He writes, "The number of meals into which the total calorie intake is divided is highly important—the *fewer* the meals, the *greater* the likelihood of obesity..." (my emphasis).

Dr. Williams not only agrees but raises an additional question. "Can eating more frequently reduce heart attacks?", he asks. "Probably. Heart attacks are often precipitated by the consumption of a heavy meal. When food is being digested, the blood is drawn to the gastrointestinal track, and the heart, especially if the arteries are corroded, is liable to get short-changed. "There have been investigations," he goes on to say, "that suggest that full meals should be replaced by more frequent consumption of less food and that this measure serves as a protection against heart attacks, and improves the functioning of appetite mechanisms."

R. What about exercise? Everybody keeps saying how important it is to staying slim but the figures don't really add up. Let's take walking, the exercise you and others spoke so enthusiastically about in the previous chapter. According to the statistics I have seen, if I walk an extra half-hour a day, then I will only burn up about 100 calories more than I would lounging around the house. Since, so I understand, a pound of fat represents 3,500 calories, it would take an awful lot of walking to make any appreciable dent in my weight.

A. Look at it this way. If you walked for an extra half-hour a day and did not increase your food intake, you would lose about 10 pounds a year. Except for a person who's really very big or very fat, 10 pounds should produce a noticeable change in appearance as well as in health.

R. However, wouldn't I eat more to make up for those calories I would be losing through walking?

A. Very likely not. As a matter of fact you might end up eating less. For reasons not fully known, physical activity seems to improve the working of the "appestat," the mechanism that turns on and shuts off our appetite. "The appestat only works well," writes Dr. John Yudkin, "with at least a moderate amount of physical activity." And Dr. Williams maintains that "Lack of exercise has a crippling effect on appestat mechanisms." Many people find that once they become physically active, their caloric intake starts to more closely match their energy expenditure. Thus, the real value of exercise comes in reducing our desire for surplus food.

R. Do you have any other suggestions for controlling weight?

A. Eat early, slowly and painfully. Eat early because some evidence indicates that the system more easily converts calories to energy earlier in the day. As the day progresses, more and more of the calories we consume may wind up as fat. As Dr. Altschule observes, "the patient who has essentially nothing for breakfast and little more for lunch but makes sure to take a large meal with meat, vegetables and dessert in the evening is an excellent candidate for obesity despite what seems not to be excessive caloric intake." Weight control begins with a proper breakfast. The same appears to hold true for good health generally. Studies of long lived people in the United States show that most of them always ate a hearty first meal of the day.

R. What about eating slowly?

A. When our stomach feels that it has had enough, it signals this feeling to the brain. The problem is that though the distance between these two organs is not great, it takes about 20 minutes for the brain to get the message. This delay prompts us to go on eating after we have a full stomach. Eating slowly can alleviate this problem. You have perhaps heard of the age-old admonition to get up from the table while you are still a bit hungry. It is good advice. Usually, you will find that in a few minutes your hunger pangs have vanished.

R. And why do you say eat "painfully"?

A. Research shows that the less pleasant the meal, the less food is likely to be consumed. Dr. Sami Hashim of Columbia University conducted an interesting experiment along these lines. He placed 24 obese and hospitalized patients on a liquid formula diet. At first the patients received the formula through a rubber tube. Though they could have as much of it as they wished, they only consumed about 400 calories a day.

After a while, the patients were given the formula in paper cups. Their average intake promptly doubled, rising to over 800 calories a day. Then Dr. Hashim and his co-workers substituted fine crystal for the paper cups. Average consumption levels now rose to more than 1,300 calories a day.

"The experiment showed," said Dr. Hashim, "that people will eat far more in a pleasant atmosphere than they will if forced to dine in austere circumstances." To those wishing to lose weight he recommends dining on paper plates and plastic spoons with no tablecloths or flowers on the table and no pleasant music in the background. For those who need even more motivation to eat less, he suggests replacing dining table chairs with uncomfortable, backless stools. Making the temperature in the dining area either too hot or too cool will also help. "If you are sitting uncomfortably, you'll be more likely to eat only what you need and leave the table rather than stick around for seconds," he says.

Dr. Hashim's advice, while probably sound, need only be considered as a last resort, to be followed if everything else fails: Eating is and should be a pleasant, social occasion. Fortunately, most people should find that simply obeying the weight control principles enunciated earlier will enable them to dispense with such

Draconian dietary measures as paper plates and hard stools.

R. Speaking of discomfort and Draconian measures, giving up cigarettes constitutes for some people the most Draconian measure of all. Yet virtually all doctors and other health practitioners believe that doing so will bring down blood pressure. Why?

A. Cigarettes tend to elevate blood pressure in many ways. The carbon monoxide in the inhaled smoke cuts down on the amount of oxygen which the heart would otherwise receive. This disrupts the heart's normal efficiency and forces it to beat faster and harder to avoid oxygen starvation. Tobacco smoke also contains cadmium whose effect on elevating blood pressure we examined in Chapter 3. Then, the nicotine in the smoke interferes with the electrical impulses which govern and guide the heart's function. Tobacco smoke also constricts the arteries which, as we saw in Chapter 1, forces the heart to pump harder. Finally, cigarette smoking is a highly addictive habit and therefore can not help but cause increased stress. Anytime a person places himself in a situation where he needs something several times a day, and becomes increasingly tense when he doesn't receive it, he is creating a lot of undue stress for himself.

For these and other reasons, cigarette smokers suffer three times as many heart attacks as non-smokers. What's more their chances of dying from such an attack are 21 times as great as those of a non-smoker.

R. Most cigarette smokers suffer intense withdrawal pains when they try to give up their habit. Is there any way in which they can avoid this agony?

A. There are ways in which they can ease the pain substantially though they can probably not eliminate it completely. For one thing, some of the nutritional steps that have been suggested for lowering blood pressure should help. Calcium and magnesium have a soothing effect on the nervous system. So, to a somewhat lesser extent, do the B vitamins. Those who are trying to kick the habit should make ample use of such nutrients. An increase in protein consumption may also help, for protein does regulate blood sugar levels.

Physical activity can also be a great aid. Now more than ever is the time to swim, walk, dance and engage in other physical activities. Many people find that suitable exercise almost automatically reduces their need and desire for tobacco. (This increased physical activity will aid the smoker in still another way as well and that is by helping him keep his weight down. As is well known, people who give up smoking tend to eat more, partly as a compensation for the oral gratification they are no longer obtaining from tobacco.)

The smoker should also try to eliminate or at least reduce the other activities in his life which he has associated with smoking. For example, if he has been accustomed to having a cigarette with a cup of coffee during the day, then he should give up the cup of coffee as well. Instead, he should drink something else or, better yet, do something entirely different.

In general, the smoker should seek to avoid events and situations which might encourage him to smoke. If invited to a cocktail party he might offer his regrets and go to a movie instead. Once the habit is safely behind him, he can start going to cocktail parties again.

Finally, there is one excellent technique available to help break any nervous habit. That technique is transcendental meditation.

R. Just what is transcendental meditation and how is it done?

A. Transcendental meditation or TM as it is called is not an occult philosophy or religion. It is essentially an effective and easy technique for relaxing the mind and body. It has been tested at the Harvard Medical School and found to be beneficial in a variety of ways. Few cigarette smokers who have practiced it for any length of time have failed to give up smoking.

R. How does one practice it?

A. It is amazingly simple. Twice a day simply sit down in a quiet spot, close your eyes and say a meaningless word to yourself. The word you choose to use doesn't really matter as long as it doesn't conjure up any particular associations. A frequent choice is the word "one." Of course, your mind will wander, but when it does, do not get upset. When you think of it, simply go back to repeating silently the word "one" or whatever word you have chosen to use. Do this for 20 minutes twice a day.

R. Is that all there is to it?

A. Almost. You should take care to do the exercise on an empty stomach. Consequently, most people who meditate do it before breakfast and again before dinner. Also, you should actually sit with your eyes closed for about 30 seconds before you start to meditate and, even more importantly, you should remain seated with your eyes closed *for at least two full minutes* after you finish meditating. During these two intervals, the 30 seconds before and the two or more minutes afterwards, you can let your mind roam at will. But even during meditation itself, don't get too frantic over getting back to repeating your meaningless word. When you think of it and when it feels comfortable to do, resume saying it to yourself. That's about all there is to it.

R. It may be quite simple to do but it does seem to require quite an investment of time. Twenty minutes twice a day plus 30 seconds before and two minutes or more afterward add up to almost an hour. Suppose you don't have the time?

A. Mary Tyler Moore, Merv Griffin and Clint Eastwood, to name some of its more notable practitioners, are all extremely busy people. Don't forget that they produce shows as well as appear in them. Yet they and numerous other celebrities find the time to meditate fully twice a day. If people such as they are not too busy then neither is any one else. Furthermore, TM tends to reduce your need for sleep so whatever time you may lose sitting in a chair and saying your "mantra," as the meaningless word is called, you will usually more than make up for by spending less time in bed.

R. What about those who simply can not or will not give up tobacco. Is there anything they can do, short of kicking the habit?

A. One thing they should carefully consider doing is exchanging cigarettes for either pipes or cigars. This includes women as well as men, for there are smaller cigars and pipes designed for them on the market. Making the switch may not be exactly painless since they will still be tempted to inhale. However, it is usually easier to switch to cigars and pipes than to give up smoking altogether. After a while, the smoker usually enjoys them more than the cigarettes he used to smoke.

Because they are usually impossible to inhale, at least on a consistent basis, and possibly because of other factors such as the absence of paper in the smoke and the differences in tobacco, cigars and pipes are nowhere near as damaging to most people as are cigarettes. Cigar and pipe smokers frequently live to advanced ages while cigarette smokers almost never do. This doesn't make such forms of tobacco usage healthful. Far from it. But, as in the case of saccharin and sugar, it is a question of choosing the lesser of two evils. And just as saccharin must be considered safer than sugar, so must pipes and cigars be judged less injurious than cigarettes.

R. We now come to stress, a subject which you have referred to frequently through the course of our discussion. One hears a great deal about stress these days. Does that mean that it is becoming an increasingly severe problem?

A. Certainly, it is becoming an increasingly noticed problem. Whether or not it is worse now than in times past can not be decisively determined. Thanks to social security, unemployment insurance, health insurance, retirement plans, trade unions and other features of modern life, we escape much of the stress which plagued our forebears. Think of the severe stress so many Americans underwent during the depression of the 1930s. If the boss looked at you the wrong way, or if any member of your family showed signs of contracting a bad illness, you immediately might start to worry about the possibility of financial destitution.

Happily, such dire situations are, for most of us, things of the past. Less happily, however, the much more comfortable conditions we enjoy today create stress situations of their own. For example, today most people can afford to take vacations. But deciding just where to go, what to do and how much to spend can create all kinds of stress. The same holds true for so many other aspects of modern life. Most of us own many more clothes than our parents possessed. As a result, simply deciding what to wear each day has become, for some people, a stressful situation. In general, the more options one has, the more decisions one has to make, and decision-making can be quite a stressful experience.

R. *How seriously does such stress affect blood pressure?*

A. It would be difficult to overstate its effect. Stress stimulates the adrenal glands which prompt the heart to pump harder. The result is a rapid rise in blood pressure. Early in 1979, a researcher at De Paul University in Illinois checked the blood pressure of 254 students before and during a final exam. Before the exam, their average was 118/58. During the exam, it registered 152/113. This represents a nearly one-third increase in the systolic or top number and an almost 100 per cent increase in the diastolic or bottom number. It vividly indicates what a stressful situation can do to blood pressure.

In another experiment, the blood pressure of a group of young adults was taken when they were calm and relaxed. Then each was individually told some bad news. The imparting of this information caused their blood pressure to rise substantially and to remain at a high level for several hours.

Finally, there is an interesting bit of research conducted by a physician named Henry I. Russek and reported in the *Journal of the American Medical Association* on October 3, 1959. Dr. Russek compared a group of 100 heart patients who were under 40 years old with a similarly aged group of patients who were suffering from other kinds of illness. He found that 91 per cent of the heart patients had undergone prolonged emotional strain associated with problems connected to their work. But in the other group of patients, only 20 per cent had experienced a similar level of stress. His findings led Dr. Russek to put emotional stress above diet, smoking, heredity, obesity and lack of physical activity as a cause of heart trouble.

R. If stress is so harmful, what can we do about it?

A. People who seem especially prone to emotional upsets would do well to consult a psychotherapist. Otherwise, they and everyone else can do a great deal to cut down on the stress that so often accompanies everyday living.

Noise is a good example of one of these stresses. Experimenters at the University of Miami found that exposing rhesus monkeys to a pattern of noise typical of a modern urban environment increased the animals' blood pressure level by over 30 per cent. These noises included things like the ring of an alarm clock, the buzz of an electric razor, the blare of an occasional car horn and so forth. Thus, avoiding such noises, even if it means wearing earmuffs while sleeping, can hold down blood pressure.

Driving to work also tends to produce stress. Studies show that commuters who take public transportation experience slower pulse rates and lower blood pressure readings in making the trip from home to office and back. Hence, taking the bus or joining a car pool will not only conserve gasoline but also health as well.

On a broader view, we would do well to routinize many of the less important aspects of our lives. For instance, take the questions of deciding what to wear, a decision which, as we saw, can produce a certain amount of stress in some people. A businessman I know has four summer suits and four winter suits. During the winter he wears one suit for a week and then automatically replaces it with the next. When the warm weather comes, he follows the same procedure with his summer suits. This simple system keeps him from ever having to expend any effort on deciding what to wear. It enables him to channel his energies into more important areas.

In general, we should try to adopt a more relaxed attitude both toward ourselves and others. We should recognize that we live in an imperfect world filled with imperfect people, and walking around in a state of perpetual indignation will do neither ourselves nor the world any good. We can always make improvements, of course, but we should avoid setting perfectionist goals for others or ourselves.

By all means, do not carry grudges. We can all expect a certain amount of dirt to be done to us as we proceed through life and focusing too much of our attention on trying to "get even" will usually prove self-defeating. President Eisenhower once said that whenever anyone did him an injustice, he would write the man's name on a piece of a paper, crumple it up and throw it in the waste paper basket. He would then promptly forget about it.

R. Isn't it possible, though, to overdo this relaxation and complacency business? If we really wanted to avoid all stress we would never get out of bed in the morning.

A. I couldn't agree more fully. Just as the absence of all blood pressure is death so would the absence of all stress be a life not much better than death. We all want, indeed we all require, some excitement and challenge. What we should do is to conserve our energies for the truly rewarding types of challenge and for the more genuinely enjoyable forms of excitement. Again attitude often plays the key role in determining whether the activity concerned will help or harm. Tennis, for example, is probably one of the least desirable forms of exercise. It is not only jerky and non rhythmic but is also extremely competitive. I have even known a professor of medicine to throw his racket to the ceiling in anger over not making a shot. No wonder so many tennis players seem to experience heart and arterial problems. Yet some people can play tennis every day and live long, healthy lives. No matter how many shots they miss, they manage to find in the game more fun than frustration.

As with tennis, so with life generally. Don't be afraid to plunge in but by all means don't overdo. Recognize and accept your limits. Set reasonable goals and be prepared for the fact that the best laid plans of mice and men often don't work out.

R. What about sex? It is often considered relaxing yet I would suppose that it raises blood pressure.

A. Blood pressure does go up doing the sex act itself. This has even been measured. Ten married male volunteers were once asked to have electrocardiograms taken during intercourse. Their blood pressure at orgasm averaged 163/81. However, the blood pressure falls soon afterwards, and since sex does promote relaxation, it probably does more benefit than harm. There is one exception, however. Married people having a secret affair will do their blood pressure a distinct disservice for the stress that such extra marital liaisons produce outweighs any of their benefits, at least as far as blood pressure control is concerned.

R. You mentioned transcendental meditation as being helpful for cigarette smokers to overcome the stress that comes in trying to break their addiction. Can TM help us deal with other kinds of stress as well?

A. It certainly can. Nearly everyone who has seriously embarked on a TM program has found himself becoming more relaxed and more able to tolerate frustration. As a matter of fact, TM has been found to lower blood pressure directly.

Dr. Herbert Benson, Director of the Hypertension Section at Boston's Beth Israel Hospital, took 36 volunteers whose blood pressure averaged 146/93.5. He had them practice meditation for several weeks and again took their blood pressure. This time it averaged out to 137/88.9, a statistically significant drop. Since the longer one meditates the better one usually does it, further reductions in blood pressure would probably occur with continued practice.

R. What about Yoga and biofeedback? Can they help reduce stress and blood pressure.

A. They certainly can. Yoga, like TM, comes from India and many of its exercises tend to induce relaxation responses similar to those which TM creates. A three-year study by three American-trained doctors at a Medical Institute in India found that Yoga could bring substantial relief from a variety of stress-related ailments. It was particularly effective when combined with TM. Interestingly enough, although all the doctors were Indians, they had never had an interest in these practices until they heard of their growing popularity in the Western world. This intrigued their curiosity and led to the studies which showed them to be of benefit.

Biofeedback is a Western and more modern technique which can also lower blood pressure. Essentially, it seeks to enable our minds to consciously control our body functions. It does require some special apparatus and some knowledge as to how to operate it. It also seems to vary greatly in its effects, at least as far as blood pressure is concerned. It works much more effectively with some people than with others. But biofeedback is certainly well worth looking into for those who are more seriously concerned with lowering blood pressure.

R. What about the Chinese practice of acupuncture? One hears a lot about acupuncture's ability to alleviate many medical problems. Can it lower blood pressure?

A. Its practitioners say it can do so. No scientific studies have apparently been done to prove it but a health writer named Betty Lee Morales says she witnessed a dramatic instance of its effectiveness. She observed a man in his 70s with a blood pressure of 200/110 being given an acupuncture treatment. Needles were placed in his feet and energized by a low-voltage electric current. After about 20 minutes, the needles were removed and the man's blood pressure was taken again. This time it registered 135/80.

R.   Are there any other specific techniques that tend to lower BP?

A. Dr. Bruno Kiveloff, the Director of Physical Medicine and Rehabilitation at the New York Infirmary, has developed a special exercise which he and his associates claim has proven remarkably effective in bringing down blood pressure. It's amazingly simple, requiring less than a minute a day. Here is what you do:

Stand in a relaxed position and then tense all your muscles. You may not be able to tense them all the first few times you try but if you can not then tense just part of your body. As you do the exercise more often, you will find yourself able to increase the tensed area until virtually all your muscles are covered. Do not, however, clench your fists or bend your elbows. Simply tighten your muscles in the position they most naturally assume.

Now, keeping your muscles tense, breathe normally for six seconds while counting out loud. Then rest for several seconds. Repeat the exercise two more times. Do this three times a day which means you will do the muscle tensing nine times daily in all. In about five to eight weeks, your blood pressure, if it is too high, should drop significantly. The most important thing, according to Dr. Kiveloff, is that you maintain *normal* breathing while you are doing it.

R.   Has this technique been scientifically studied?

A. Dr. Kiveloff published a study of his own in the *Journal of the American Geriatrics Society* in 1971. His test group consisted of 22 people, seven of whom had normal blood pressure while the other 15 had hypertension. Of the 15 with hypertension, seven were taking drugs to control it.

The exercise had no effect on those with normal BP. It reduced by up to 18 per cent the BP of those taking drugs. For those not taking drugs, the reductions ranged up to 25 and 27 per cent. It apparently works well, providing a person with high blood pressure sticks with it long enough and remembers to do the exercises three times a day.

R. We have certainly covered a lot of ground in this chapter. Since it is the last one before the summing up, are there any other things you can recommend for blood pressure control?

A. Yes. Personal integrity.

R. Integrity? I thought blood pressure control was a physical problem not a philosophical one. What does an ethical concern such as integrity have to do with it?

A. Every time we lie or deceive, we subject ourselves to stress. The whole principle of the lie detector is based on this. Lie detectors, when operated by fully trained people, are virtually impossible for even the most astute liars to beat. That's because all of us, even the least praiseworthy among us, apparently do not find lying natural.

The same holds true for any other practices that may impair our integrity. Such practices create some degree of stress in nearly all of us and we would do well to give them up. The more we behave as we think people should behave, the more we will be able to avoid added stress and strain.

The ancient Greeks believed that virtue was its own reward. Modern science is showing that they knew what they were talking about.

CHAPTER 8

The Added Bonus

R. My first question, naturally, has to do with the title of this chapter. What is the added bonus?

A. It would be better, perhaps, to talk of added bonuses. It refers to the fact that virtually all the steps one should take to lower blood pressure will also contribute to a longer, healthier life in other ways, as well.

R. That's certainly good to know. And, as a matter of fact, you have from time to time touched on some of these added advantages in your recommendations. But let's go through the list again and this time point out just what else we can expect from each item. You have mentioned so many things that reviewing them all will also help to keep them in mind.

A. Fine. However, I will not be able to state *all* the fringe benefits which a regimen designed to lower blood pressure will produce. That would take several books. I will only try to touch on some of the most important.

Let us begin with those two critical minerals, salt and potassium. Salt, in excess of a minimum amount, can cause other calamities besides HBP. For years some doctors suspected salt of causing or contributing to cancer as well. Then, in the mid 1970s, the World Health Organization did a study confirming this suspicion. The study, which was carried out in Japan, showed a high correlation between cancer and salt consumption.

Salt has also been implicated in a variety of other ailments. They include migraine headaches and kidney problems. There is little doubt that the average American could do his overall health a great deal of good by drastically cutting down on salt.

Potassium, on the other hand, can confer many benefits besides simply counteracting the effects of salt. It helps prevent muscle weakness and also helps transport vitamins to the cells of the body. Vitamin C, for example, seems to work more effectively when taken in the form of a potassium compound. Potassium's ability to protect the heart itself was already noted earlier. Autopsies on people who have died of heart attacks have shown that their hearts contained much less potassium than the hearts of those who have died from other causes.

R. What about the other minerals you mentioned, such as calcium, magnesium, zinc, chromium and selenium?

A. They all have extra benefits to bestow. Calcium, as most everybody knows, is vital for the bones and teeth. And as I sought to point out in Chapter 3, it is a mineral we need for this purpose as long as we live. Its relationship to human health continues to remain high from the cradle to the grave.

It would also be difficult to overstate magnesium's role in human health. It acts with calcium in a variety of ways. For example, although a high calcium intake can benefit the teeth, it will fail to do so unless a sufficient supply of magnesium is present. In addition, magnesium seems to provide some protection against cancer. Animals placed on magnesium-deficient diets quickly develop cancerous growths.

Zinc, as also noted earlier, plays a great role in helping us combat a number of medical problems, such as ulcers, prostatitis, burns and even cancer. More minor problems such as a diminished sense of smell, premature graying of the hair and skin eruptions such as acne have been alleviated with zinc.

Chromium has been found to improve the system's capacity to cope with sugar. I believe I touched on this earlier but it needs to be underscored for few doctors have taken the trouble to read the research concerning it. Keep in mind that most people experience some difficulties in blood sugar regulation as they grow older. Chromium can therefore be of use to nearly all of us in this respect. However, it is, of course, most beneficial to those who have diabetes or who believe they are susceptible to diabetes.

Selenium has given rise to some of the more sensational research regarding trace minerals in recent years. Besides helping to bring down blood pressure and to protect the heart, it also appears to help us ward off cancer as well. There have been several experiments with animals which lead to this conclusion. As for its effect on cancer in human beings, there is a rather startling statistical study that was carried out by the Cleveland Clinic Foundation. Researchers at the foundation examined cancer rates and soil selenium content in some 150 metropolitan areas that were roughly comparable in size. They found that the incidence of cancer correlated *inversely* with the amount of selenium in the soil. The lowest cancer rate was found in Rapid City, South Dakota whose soil had the highest selenium content. The highest cancer rate turned up in Lima, Ohio, which had the lowest amount of selenium in its soil.

R. What about the vitamins you recommended? What added bonuses do they offer?

A. Again, we could fill up a whole book, and it would be a big one at that, in trying to list them all. I can only touch on a few.

Let us start with vitamin C. We now have pretty good, indeed I would say excellent, evidence that vitamin C bolsters the body's immune system. This is what most of us call "resistance," as when we speak of our ability to fight off colds and other such illnesses. Wounds, for example, heal much more rapidly when there is enough vitamin C in the system. A good deal of research has arisen concerning vitamin C's ability to help prevent colds. This research has produced varying results but the best of it, namely a scrupulously thorough study conducted by three physicians at the University of Toronto Medical School vindicated the vitamin's supporters. The study was done with over 800 students and it revealed that those students who took 1,000 milligrams of vitamin C a day suffered 30 per cent fewer colds. A heavier daily dosage might have provided even greater protection.

This Toronto experiment also produced another noteworthy finding. Those students receiving the vitamin C also experienced a surprisingly sharp drop in the incidence of other forms of illness. This confirms other research showing vitamin C to be helpful in alleviating allergies, prickly heat, hepatitis and a host of medical predicaments.

Perhaps the most exciting development concerning vitamin C concerns its potential for combatting cancer. In the early 1970s several Scottish physicians gave 10,000 milligrams of the vitamin a day to 50 cancer patients. These were all terminal cases, and were now considered to be beyond any other form of medical care. The progress of their illness was compared with the case records of another 1,000 patients who had had roughly similar cancers that were at the same stage of growth. The physicians found that the 50 who received the vitamin C lived, on the average, more than *four times longer* than did the comparison group. As a matter of fact, some of these patients staged a complete recovery and are living today. (None of the patients whose cases had been used for comparison had proven to be so fortunate.)

R. You make vitamin C sound like some sort of all-purpose miracle drug.

A. It probably represents one of the great medical breakthroughs of our time. However, you must remember that it works largely through boosting and buttressing the immune system. It will not cure illnesses by itself but will simply give the system a better chance of overcoming them. Often it is most effective when used either as a preventive or as an adjunct to more conventional medical therapy. It does not give us a magic cure-all but it does help our bodies cope with medical calamities.

Let me give you an example. Taking 2,000 milligrams of vitamin C every day will greatly increase your resistance to colds. But if, for instance, you overwork and fail to get enough sleep, you may still come down with the sniffles or even the flu. It depends on how strong your resistance was to begin with and how much strain it has been subjected to. What can be said is that, with sufficient vitamin C, your resistance will hold out longer and recover faster.

R. What about the other vitamins?

A. They too can accomplish much in improving all around health. The B vitamins help the nerves as well as the immune system. Vitamin E has enabled laboratory animals to survive a degree of air pollution that would otherwise have killed them. Researchers at MIT have found vitamin A highly effective in helping test animals resist certain kinds of induced cancers.

Many of these vitamins have been found to lengthen life. A biochemist at Columbia increased the life span of rats by more than 10 per cent by adding extra amounts of vitamin A to their diet. Dr. Roger Williams increased the life span of rats by almost 20 per cent through giving them supplemental amounts of pantothenic acid, a B vitamin. Vitamin E has been tested many times for its effect on the aging process and has been found helpful in slowing it down.

Bear in mind that some of the nation's top physicians now take vitamin supplements. (See Chapter 4 for their names.) Mention their names to your own doctor the next time he insists that a "balanced" diet supplies all the vitamins one needs, and that only a "health nut" would take extra amounts.

R. What about the good and bad foods? Are they good and bad for other reasons besides their effect on blood pressure?

A. They most assuredly are. Garlic, to take the prime example from among the good ones, is undoubtedly one of the most healthful plants in existence. In Russia doctors even prescribe it for the flu. One truly notable but, unfortunately, little noticed experiment concerning garlic and its uses was conducted at Western Reserve University in 1957. Two biochemists found that feeding test animals garlic would greatly increase their resistance to cancer-causing chemicals.

If garlic can help fortify us against cancer then meat and sugar, to take the two prime examples from among the bad foods, can do the opposite. You may recall that a comparison between Seventh-Day Adventists and Mormons showed that the largely non-meat eating Adventists had lower blood pressure. Another study has shown that they have a lower cancer rate as well. As for sugar, three different studies have distinctly and definitively demonstrated that this sweetener weakens the immune system. And in 1978 the British Cancer Institute revealed the results of research showing sugar to be the number one dietary component in breast cancer. (Fat placed second while protein took third place on the list of nutritional culprits responsible for this malady.)

R. From what you say it would seem that, forgetting its effect on blood pressure and heart problems, sugar is more cancer-causing than saccharin?

A. Exactly. The great tragedy is that we have raised

so little hue and cry about sugar and so much on its less harmful substitutes.

R. The study that you just mentioned cited fat as the second most important dietary component in breast cancer. Would this be true of other types of cancer as well? And what kinds of fat are likely to be more cancer-causing, animal fat or vegetable fat?

A. We have an abundance of evidence linking fat to various forms of cancer. As to which kinds of fat are the most perilous for human health, there appears to be no question that vegetable fat can claim this dubious distinction. This at least is true when such fat has been heated or hydrogenated.

In a study carried out at the University of Nebraska some years ago, one group of mice were fed heated corn oil while another group were given heated butter. Over a 40-month period none of the animals receiving the butter showed any sign of undue injury. But *every one of the animals receiving the heated corn oil developed cancerous tumors*.

More recently a research team at the University of Maryland did a survey of cancer rates as related to changes in diet over the years. The researchers found that, from 1909 to 1972, the average American's consumption of vegetable fat more than doubled. During the same time, the average intake of animal fat slightly declined. This increase in vegetable fat consumption was accompanied by substantial increases in breast and bowel-colon cancer. This fact plus other data led the team's leader, Dr. Mark Keeney, to conclude that "processed oils and not animal fats are the culprit in breast and colon cancer." Note his use of the word "processed." In the natural form, such oils can play quite a different role.

At Texas A&M University, Dr. Randall Wood, a Professor of Biochemistry with 15 years experience in researching cancer, agrees with this finding. Says Dr. Wood, "We have indications that partially hydrogenated vegetable fats may in fact . . . cause or contribute to production of cancer cells in the body."

For a final bit of proof—and this does not by any means exhaust all the available evidence—let us take a second look at the Veteran's hospital experiment that we examined in Chapter 6. As you may recall, it was found that although the veterans eating the diet high in polyunsaturates suffered fewer fatal heart attacks, this group also contained far fewer cigarette smokers and older veterans than did the group eating the standard American diet. Well, further follow-up showed that the vegetable fat-eating group experienced a much high cancer rate. When you take into account its smaller percentage of cigarette smokers and older veterans, this increased number of cancer deaths seems truly alarming.

R. Can heated and/or processed vegetable oils cause any other ailments or afflictions?

A. They certainly can. To return once again to the veteran's hospital experiment, the follow-up study further disclosed that the group which ate a lot of unsaturates also experienced 19 per cent more cases of gallstones.

In another study done in California, two physicians examined 800 patients over seven years. They found that those who consumed a lot of polyunsaturates appeared to age much more rapidly. Some 78 per cent of those whose diets included high amounts of polyunsaturates looked far older than their years. Commented one of the physicians, Dr. Calvan O. Griffiths, Jr., "there is no question that overeating polyunsaturates leads to wrinkles, crow's feet and other visible signs of premature aging." Dr. Griffiths, by the way, is a former professor of surgery at the University of California.

At the other geographical end of the country, Dr. Joseph Vitale, of the Boston University School of Medicine, presents other grounds for indicting such fats. He has found that putting people on diets high in polyunsaturates tends to damage and even destroy their immunization system. He has found that cancer patients who switched to such diets lost their natural defenses against the disease. However, in both these studies, no distinction was made as far as I know between the natural and processed forms of fat. And most unsaturated fat in the current American diet has been processed.

R. But you did say that a certain amount of unsaturated fat was useful, even perhaps necessary, to human health.

A. That's true. They do a much better job than the saturated fats in supplying certain acids which the system needs. They also furnish other nourishing nutrients. However, they best perform this function when they have *not* been subjected to heat or other forms of processing.

One reason why unprocessed and unheated unsaturates are not only less dangerous but even health-building is that in their natural state they contain valuable amounts of vitamin E. This vitamin can protect the body against much, perhaps most, of the injury which these fats can cause. The way that it does so lies beyond the scope of a book such as this but the fact that it does so is widely accepted. At least two respected research physicians, Dr. T. W. Anderson of the University of Toronto and Dr. Benham Harman of the University of Nebraska, have published work attesting to this and virtually all other researchers in the field agree with them. Even such a conservative establishment nutritionist as the newspaper columnist Jean Mayer has grudgingly conceded that a diet high in polyunsaturates could benefit from vitamin E supplementation.

R. What about saturated fats? Earlier you said that they too could harm the heart. Do they also injure health in other ways?

A. Yes. They may cause difficulties with digestion and aggravate weight problems. And like the unsaturates, they too can cause or contribute to such ailments as gallstones and cancer. As regards this latter illness, Dr. John Berg of the University of Iowa has claimed that animal fats upset the body's hormonal balance, producing, in his words, "the same effect that one would obtain running a diesel engine on high octane fuel." This, so he told a conference sponsored by the National Cancer Institute, can lead to cancer.

An interesting experiment which perhaps sums up well the whole situation was conducted at the Boston University School of Medicine. Their results were revealed in 1977. One group of rats was raised on a diet high in vegetable fats, which were probably of the processed kind, another group was given a diet high in animal fats; and a third group was fed a diet low in both kinds of fat. All of the animals were then injected with a cancer-causing chemical.

All of the processed vegetable oil eaters contracted

cancer while 85 per cent of the animal fat eaters developed the disease. But only 50 per cent of those on the low-fat diet came down with malignant tumors.

R. However, you did quote Dr. Williams as saying that butterfat does aid the system in synthesizing vitamin B6. Does this mean that it is meat fat and not dairy fat which is most to be shunned?

A. Right. Fatty meats should have a low place on the menu of every health-conscious person. And don't forget that beef contains almost as much fat as most kinds of pork, although neither should be heavily consumed. Chicken and turkey have the lowest fat content of all meats and are the safest to eat.

R. But didn't primitive man eat a lot of wild game? Did he suffer a great deal from the health problems you attribute to animal fats?

A. The meat of wild animals contains much less fat than that of domestic ones. Cows and pigs today are even fed diets especially designed to make them fat. Also, primitive man ate much if not most of his meat raw. In doing so he ingested a good deal of vitamin B6 along with it. Some provocative research has recently come to light pointing up the vitamin's protective value in relation to meat. This research largely focuses on the ways in which vitamin B6 helps the system metabolize meat protein but the possibility definitely exists that it helps us handle meat fats as well.

Two MIT scientists wrote a most interesting article on this subject for the May, 1979 issue of *The Atlantic*. I strongly urge everyone to read it. They claim that B6 enables the body to protect itself from the cholesterol-causing components present in protein. They maintain that Eskimos do not develop arteriosclerosis despite their high consumption of animal flesh because they eat so much of it raw, and in this form it contains substantial amounts of vitamin B6. Although their data related to protein, not fat, and to heart-related illnesses only, still their report is not irrelevant to what we have just been discussing. It also may shed new light on the possible dangers of the high-protein diet which we examined in discussing weight control. It may well be that too much protein *in the absence of sufficient vitamin B6* constitutes the problem.

R. What about the high fiber diet which you proposed as an alternative to the high-protein diet as a way of keeping down weight? Does it offer any supplementary health benefits?

A. It certainly does. First of all, high-fiber foods are usually rich in many vitamins, minerals and other desirable nutrients. More importantly, fibrous foods help our digestive systems work more efficiently. In doing so they enable us to get rid of waste products before they putrefy and become toxic to the system. They help us avoid straining during bowel movements. Such straining can cause hemorrhoids, varicose veins and even appendicitis. Finally, high fiber diets appear to protect those who consume them from bowel-colon cancer. Don't forget that next to lung cancer, bowel-colon malignancy is the country's second greatest cause of cancer death.

R. Giving up cigarette smoking would pretty much free us from the danger of the biggest cancer killer, would it not?

A. Pretty much. About 90 per cent of all lung cancer cases are connected to tobacco. Cigarette smoking can also cause emphysema and other bronchial conditions. Furthermore, inhaling cigarette smoke destroys vitamin C in the body and we have seen how vital a role this vitamin plays in keeping us healthy.

R. That leaves only stress to consider.

A. Stress is destructive to our systems in many ways. It increases the pulse rate, overstimulates our hormonal system and depletes the body of vitamin C. It puts a great strain on our immunization system thereby making us more susceptible to all kinds of medical maladies.

R. Well, I guess that just about completes this list. And it does seem that the recommendations you have made earlier for lowering blood pressure are worth the sacrifices they entail.

A. Sacrifices? Where did you get this word "sacrifices?" Changes, yes, but sacrifices? Ha.dly. If you follow the do's and don'ts for lowering blood pressure you will actually enjoy eating more than you did before. Losing weight and giving up cigarettes may be painful at first but eventually you will enjoy those alterations in your life as well. Certainly, reducing stress should logically leave one more contented and you will find that it does. People who start practicing TM soon discover that, in addition to its other benefits, it also quite simply makes them happier.

Health and happiness, in other words, are scarcely conflicting or contradictory goals. On the contrary, they go hand-in-hand together. Try it and see.

Afterword

Dear R.,

Between the time this book was written and the time it went to the printer, some new developments occurred in the increasingly active field of health. Happily, these developments generally supported and strengthened points made in the original manuscript. For example in the Spring of 1980 the Food and Nutrition Board finally conceded that the claims made for unsaturated fats, and the charges made against eggs, were for the most part, without any reliable basis in fact. Many cardiologists protested this finding, but they could produce no truly solid evidence to refute it.

A few months later *Executive Health* reported some preliminary results from a sweeping 20-year study on health which the American Cancer Society had just concluded. The study showed that egg-eaters suffered fewer heart attacks and strokes, on the average, than those who largely abstained from eggs. It did show that men who exercise suffer less heart disease and fewer strokes, but, like similar studies in the past, it indicated that the greatest gain comes from moderate exercise. Also, no effort was apparently made to isolate the other differences between the exercise and non-exercise groups that may have influenced the results such as smoking, heavy drinking, over-eating, etc.

One possible help in blood pressure control which

is hardly new but which I was unaware of at the time I wrote the preceding chapters is chiropractic. Many chiropractors claim that through manipulation of the spine and related parts of the body they can reduce blood pressure. Dr. Michael J. Butler, a Boston chiropractor, says he has found that many high blood pressure sufferers are also suffering from a dropped sacrum, and that raising the sacrum, which is a bone at the base of the spine, often lowers their blood pressure.

Some chiropractors give the HBP patients herbal diuretics which, they maintain, work much more effectively than the drugs prescribed by medical doctors. These herbal medicines also do not generate the adverse side effects which so frequently accompany regular blood pressure drugs. Dr. Bruce Josefek, another Boston chiropractor, says he has received excellent results from a compound consisting of uva ursi and buchu extracts.

I cannot vouch for any of these remedies. But I can vouch for the effectiveness of chiropractic in treating a good many ills. So, if you feel you need additional help in controlling your blood pressure, why not consult a good chiropractor? Since they do not use surgery or drugs they can rarely do anyone any harm. And many have found them to be beneficial indeed.

Selected
Bibliography

Adams, Ruth and Murray, Frank. *Body, Mind and the B Vitamins*. Foreword by Abram Hoffer, M.D. (N.Y.: Larchmont), 1972.

Adams, Ruth and Murray, Frank. *Health Foods* (N.Y.: Larchmont), 1975. Foreword by S. Marshall Fram, M.D.

Adams, Ruth and Murray, Frank. *Minerals: Kill or Cure?* Foreword by Harvey M. Ross, M.D. (N.Y.: Larchmont), 1974.

Altschule, Mark D., M.D. "How Much Do You Know That Isn't So About Saturated vs. Unsaturated Fats?" *Executive Health* 10, (1974).

Altschule, Mark D., M.D. "The Much-Maligned Egg." *Executive Health* Volume X, Number 8.

Altschule, Mark D., M.D. *Nutritional Factors in General Medicine*. (Springfield, Illinois: Charles C. Thomas), 1978.

Benson, Herbert, M.D. *The Relaxation Response*. (N.Y.: William Morrow), 1975.

Bricklin, Mark. *The Practical Encyclopedia of Natural Healing*. (Emmaus, Pa.: Rodale Press), 1976.

Clark, Linda. *Handbook of Natural Remedies for Common Ailments*. (N.Y.: Pocket Books), 1976.

Coca, Arthur F., M.D. *The Pulse Test*. (N.Y.: Lyle Stuart) Revised edition, 1967.

Frank, Benjamin S., M.D. *Dr. Frank's No-Aging Diet*. (N.Y.: Dial Press), 1976.

Hrachovec, Josef P., M.D., D.Sc. *Keeping Young and Living Longer*. (Los Angeles: Sherbourne Press), 1972.

Mességué, Maurice. *C'est la Nature Qui a Raison*. (Paris: Robert Laffort), 1972.

Murray, Frank. *Program Your Heart For Health*. (N.Y.: Larchmont), 1977. Foreword by Michael Walczak, M.D. Introduction by E. Cheraskin, M.D.

Passwater, Richard, Ph.D. *Supernutrition for Healthy Hearts*. (N.Y.: Jove), 1977.

Pfeiffer, Carl C., M.D. *Zinc and Other Micro-Nutrients*. (New Canaan, Conn.: Keats Publishing), 1978.

Selye, Hans, M.D. *The Stress of Life*. (N.Y.: McGraw-Hill), 1976.

Wade, Carlson. *Hypertension (High Blood Pressure) and Your Diet*. (New Canaan, Conn.: Keats Publishing, Inc.), 1975.

Williams, Roger J., Ph.D. *Nutrition Against Disease*. (N.Y.: Bantam), 1973.

Yudkin, John, M.D. *Sweet and Dangerous*. (N.Y.: Peter H. Wyden, Inc.), 1972.

Here is the Potassium Content of Some Common Foods, Along with the Sodium Content:

Foods	Sodium in 1 serving of 100 grams	Potassium in 1 serving of 100 grams
Almonds	2.0	690
Brazil nuts	0.8	650
Filberts	0.8	560
Peanuts	0.8	740
Walnuts	2.0	450
Apples	0.1	68
Apricots	0.5	440
Bananas	0.1	400
Cherries	1.0	280
Oranges	0.2	170
Peaches	0.1	180
Plums	0.1	140
Strawberries	0.7	180
Barley	3.0	160
Corn	0.4	290
Oats	2.0	340
Rice	0.8	100
Wheat	2.0	430
Beans, snap	0.8	300
Lima beans	1.0	700
Navy beans, dry	0.9	1,300
Fresh peas	0.9	380
Broccoli	16.0	400
Cabbage	5.0	230
Cauliflower	24.0	400
Lettuce	12.0	140
Spinach	190.0	790
Celery	110.0	300
Beets	110.0	350
Carrots	31.0	410
Potatoes	0.6	410
Turnips	5.0	260
Whole eggs	14.0	130
Whole milk	51.0	140
Beef	53.0	380

Foods	Sodium in 1 serving of 100 grams	Potassium in 1 serving of 100 grams
Chicken	110.0	250
Fish	60.0	360
Lamb	110.0	340
Turkey	92.0	310

Foods with High Salt Content

Bacon
Beef, corned
Beef, dried
Bouillon cubes
Breads,
  commercial
Catsup
Caviar
Cheese
Codfish, salted
Cereals,
  commercial

Crackers,
  commercial
Ham
Herring, smoked
Hot dogs
Luncheon meats
Mustard
Olives
Pickles

Pizza
Popcorn, salted
Potato chips
Salad dressings,
  commercial
Salt pork
Salted nuts
Sausage
Soups, canned

Because some products vary considerably in sodium content, the following table gives representative values. Sodium values shown reflect current processing practices and typical product formulas. If these practices and formulas are changed, sodium values may change also.

Values given in the table are for unsalted products, unless specified. Cooked items have been prepared using unsalted water, even though the manufacturers' instructions may call for salt. Canned vegetable values are for total can contents of solids and liquids. The values reported are for common household measures of the foods and include metric equivalents.

Some labels may express sodium content in grams or milligrams. Here's how to convert these measurements and also how to measure the amount of sodium in salt.

Sodium Content of Food

Beverages and Fruit Juices

Food	Portion	Weight (grams)	Sodium (milli-grams)
Alcoholic:			
Beer	12 fl oz	360	25
Gin, rum, whiskey	2 fl oz	60	1
Wine:			
Red:			
Domestic	4 fl oz	120	12
Imported	4 fl oz	120	6
Sherry	4 fl oz	120	14
White:			
Domestic	4 fl oz	120	19
Imported	4 fl oz	120	2

Source: "The Sodium Content of Your Food," by Anne C. Marsh, Ruth N. Klippstein and Sybil D. Kaplan, Home and Garden Bulletin No. 233, USDA, August, 1980.

Anne C. Marsh is a Nutrition Analyst with the Consumer Nutrition Center, SEA, USDA, Washington, D. C.; Ruth N. Klippstein is Professor, Division of Nutritional Sciences, Cornell University, Ithaca, N. Y.; and Sybil D. Kaplan is a Cooperative Extension Specialist, University of Rhode Island, Kingston, R. I.

Food	Portion	Weight (grams)	Sodium (milligrams)
Breakfast drink, instant:			
Grape	8 fl oz	240	0
Citrus fruits	8 fl oz	240	14
Carbonated:			
Club soda	8 fl oz	240	39
Cola:			
Regular	8 fl oz	240	16
Low calorie	8 fl oz	240	21
Fruit flavored:			
Regular	8 fl oz	240	34
Low calorie	8 fl oz	240	46
Ginger ale	8 fl oz	240	13
Root beer	8 fl oz	240	24
Cocoa mix, water added	8 fl oz	240	232
Coffee:			
Brewed	8 fl oz	240	2
Instant:			
Regular	8 fl oz	240	1
Decaffeinated	8 fl oz	240	1
With chicory	8 fl oz	240	7
With flavorings	8 fl oz	240	124
Substitute	8 fl oz	240	3
Fruit drinks, canned:			
Apple	8 fl oz	240	16
Cranberry juice cocktail	8 fl oz	240	4
Grape	8 fl oz	240	1
Lemonade	8 fl oz	240	60
Orange	8 fl oz	240	77
Pineapple-grapefruit	8 fl oz	240	80
Fruit drinks, dehydrated, reconstituted:			
Sweetened:			
Lemonade	8 fl oz	240	50
Orange	8 fl oz	240	35
Other fruit	8 fl oz	240	0
Unsweetened, all flavors	8 fl oz	240	0
Fruit juices:			
Apple cider or juice	1 cup	248	5
Apricot nectar	1 cup	251	9

167

Food	Portion	Weight (grams)	Sodium (milli-grams)

Citrus:

    Grapefruit juice:

Food	Portion	Weight (grams)	Sodium (milli-grams)
Canned	1 cup	250	4
Frozen, diluted	1 cup	247	5
Lemon or lime juice:			
Canned	1 cup	244	2
Frozen, diluted	1 cup	248	4
Orange juice:			
Canned	1 cup	249	5
Frozen, diluted	1 cup	249	5
Tangerine juice	1 cup	249	2
Grape juice, bottled	1 cup	253	8
Peach nectar	1 cup	249	10
Pear nectar	1 cup	250	8
Pineapple juice	1 cup	250	5
Prune juice	1 cup	256	5
Mineral water, imported	8 fl oz	240	42
Tea:			
Hot:			
Brewed	8 fl oz	240	1
Instant	8 fl oz	240	2
Iced:			
Canned	8 fl oz	240	9
Powdered, lemon flavored:			
Sugar sweetened	8 fl oz	240	1
Low calorie	8 fl oz	240	15
Thirst quencher	8 fl oz	240	140

Dairy Products

Cheese:

Food	Portion	Weight (grams)	Sodium (milli-grams)
Natural:			
Blue	1 oz	28	396
Brick	1 oz	28	159
Brie	1 oz	28	178
Camembert	1 oz	28	239
Cheddar:			
Regular	1 oz	28	176
Low sodium	1 oz	28	6

Food	Portion	Weight (grams)	Sodium (milligrams)
Colby	1 oz	28	171
Cottage:			
Regular and lowfat	4 oz	113	457
Dry curd, unsalted	4 oz	113	14
Cream	1 oz	28	84
Edam	1 oz	28	274
Feta	1 oz	28	316
Gouda	1 oz	28	232
Gruyere	1 oz	28	95
Limburger	1 oz	28	227
Monterey	1 oz	28	152
Mozzarella, from:			
Whole milk	1 oz	28	106
Part skim milk	1 oz	28	132
Muenster	1 oz	28	178
Neufchatel	1 oz	28	113
Parmesan:			
Grated	1 oz	28	528
Hard	1 oz	28	454
Provolone	1 oz	28	248
Ricotta, made with:			
Whole milk	½ cup	124	104
Part skim milk	½ cup	124	155
Roquefort	1 oz	28	513
Swiss	1 oz	28	74
Tilsit	1 oz	28	213
Pasteurized processed cheese:			
American	1 oz	28	406
Low sodium	1 oz	28	2
Swiss	1 oz	28	388
Cheese food:			
American	1 oz	28	337
Swiss	1 oz	28	440
Cheese spread:			
American	1 oz	28	381
Cream, sweet:			
Fluid, all types	1 tbsp	15	6
Whipped	1 tbsp	3	4
Cream, sour, cultured	1 tbsp	12	6

Food	Portion	Weight (grams)	Sodium (milligrams)
Cream products, imitation:			
Sweet:			
Coffee whitener:			
Liquid	1 tbsp	15	12
Powdered	1 tbsp	6	12
Whipped Topping	1 tbsp	4	2
Sour, cultured	1 oz	28	29
Milk:			
Fluid:			
Whole and lowfat	1 cup	244	122
Whole, low sodium	1 cup	244	6
Buttermilk, cultured:			
Salted	1 cup	245	257
Unsalted	1 cup	245	122
Canned:			
Evaporated:			
Whole	1 cup	252	266
Skim	1 cup	255	294
Sweetened, condensed	1 cup	306	389
Dry:			
Nonfat:			
Regular	½ cup	60	322
Instantized	1 cup	68	373
Buttermilk	½ cup	60	310
Milk beverages:			
Chocolate	1 cup	250	149
Cocoa, hot	1 cup	250	123
Eggnog	1 cup	254	138
Malted:			
Natural flavor	1 cup	265	215
Chocolate flavor	1 cup	265	168
Shakes, thick:			
Chocolate or vanilla	1 shake	306	317
Milk desserts, frozen			
Ice cream:			
Chocolate	1 cup	133	75
Custard, French	1 cup	133	84
Strawberry	1 cup	133	77

Food	Portion	Weight (grams)	Sodium (milligrams)
Vanilla:			
French, softserve	1 cup	173	153
Hardened	1 cup	140	112
Ice milk:			
Vanilla:			
Hardened	1 cup	131	105
Soft serve	1 cup	175	163
Novelty products:			
Bars:			
Fudge	1 bar	73	54
Orange cream	1 bar	66	27
Vanilla, chocolate coated:			
Ice cream	1 bar	47	24
Ice milk	1 bar	50	31
Cones, vanilla, chocolate coated	1 small	71	64
Sandwich	1 sandwich	62	92
Sherbet, orange	1 cup	193	89
Milk desserts, other:			
Custard, baked	1 cup	265	209
Puddings:			
Butterscotch:			
Regular, whole milk	½ cup	148	245
Instant, whole milk	½ cup	149	445
LoCal, skim milk	½ cup	130	130
Ready-to-serve	1 can	142	290
Chocolate:			
Home recipe	½ cup	130	73
Regular, whole milk	½ cup	148	195
Instant, whole milk	½ cup	149	470
LoCal, skim milk	½ cup	130	80
Ready-to-serve	1 can	142	262
Vanilla:			
Home recipe	½ cup	128	83
Regular, whole milk	½ cup	148	200
Instant, whole milk	½ cup	149	400
LoCal, skim milk	½ cup	130	115
Ready-to-serve	1 can	142	279
Tapioca, cooked	½ cup	145	130

171

Food	Portion	Weight (grams)	Sodium (milligrams)
Yogurt:			
Plain:			
Regular	8 oz	227	105
Lowfat	8 oz	227	159
Skim milk	8 oz	227	174
With fruit	8 oz	227	133

Eggs, Fish, Shellfish, Meat, Poultry, and Related Products

Food	Portion	Weight (grams)	Sodium (milligrams)
Eggs:			
Whole	1 egg	50	59
White	1 white	33	50
Yolk	1 yolk	17	9
Substitute, frozen	¼ cup	60	120
Fish:			
Bass, black sea, raw	3 oz	85	57
Bluefish:			
Baked with butter	3 oz	85	87
Breaded, fried	3 oz	85	123
Bonito, canned	3 oz	85	437
Catfish, raw	3 oz	85	50
Cod, broiled with butter	3 oz	85	93
Eel, raw	3 oz	85	67
Flounder (includes sole and other flat fish) baked with butter	3 oz	85	201
Haddock, breaded, fried	3 oz	85	150
Halibut, broiled with butter	3 oz	85	114
Herring, smoked	3 oz	85	5,234
Lingcod, raw	3 oz	85	50
Mackerel, raw	3 oz	85	40
Mullet, breaded, fried	3 oz	85	83
Ocean perch, fried	3 oz	85	128
Pollock, creamed	3 oz	85	94
Pompano, cooked	3 oz	85	48
Rockfish, ovensteamed	3 oz	85	57

Food	Portion	Weight (grams)	Sodium (milligrams)
Salmon:			
Broiled with butter	3 oz	85	99
Canned:			
Salt added:			
Pink	3 oz	85	443
Red	3 oz	85	329
Silver	3 oz	85	298
Without salt added	3 oz	85	41
Sardines, canned:			
Drained	3 oz	85	552
In tomato sauce	3 oz	85	338
Shad, baked with butter	3 oz	85	66
Snapper, raw	3 oz	85	56
Trout, lake, raw	3 oz	85	67
Tuna, canned:			
Light meat, chunk:			
Oil pack	3 oz	85	303
Water pack	3 oz	85	288
Grated	3 oz	85	246
White meat (Albacore)			
Chunk, low sodium	3 oz	85	34
Solid:			
Oil pack	3 oz	85	384
Water pack	3 oz	85	309
Shellfish:			
Clams, raw:			
Hard	3 oz	85	174
Soft	3 oz	85	30
Crab:			
Canned, drained	3 oz	85	425
Steamed	3 oz	85	314
Lobster, boiled	3 oz	85	212
Mussels, raw	3 oz	85	243
Oysters:			
Raw	3 oz	85	113
Fried	3 oz	85	174
Frozen	3 oz	85	323

Food	Portion	Weight (grams)	Sodium (milligrams)
Scallops:			
Raw	3 oz	85	217
Steamed	3 oz	85	225
Shrimp:			
Raw	3 oz	85	137
Fried	3 oz	85	159
Canned	3 oz	85	1,955
Meat:			
Beef			
Cooked, lean	3 oz	85	55
Corned:			
Cooked	3 oz	85	802
Canned	3 oz	85	893
Dried, chipped	1 oz	28	1,219
Lamb, cooked, lean	3 oz	85	58
Pork:			
Cured:			
Bacon:			
Cooked	2 slices	14	274
Canadian	1 slice	28	394
Ham	3 oz	85	1,114
Salt pork, raw	1 oz	28	399
Fresh, cooked, lean	3 oz	85	59
Veal, cooked, lean	3 oz	85	69
Organ meats:			
Brain, raw	1 oz	28	35
Gizzard, poultry, simmered	1 oz	28	17
Heart:			
Beef, braised	1 oz	28	29
Calf, braised	1 oz	28	32
Poultry, simmered	1 oz	28	14
Kidney, beef, braised	1 oz	28	71
Liver:			
Calf, fried	1 oz	28	33
Pork, simmered	1 oz	28	14
Poultry, simmered	1 oz	28	16
Sweetbreads, calf, cooked	1 oz	28	32
Tongue, beef, braised	1 oz	28	17
Tripe:			
Commercial	1 oz	28	13

Food	Portion	Weight (grams)	Sodium (milligrams)
Poultry and game:			
Chicken, roasted:			
Breast with skin	½ breast	98	69
Drumstick with skin	1 drumstick	52	47
Products:			
Canned	1 5-oz can	142	714
Frankfurter	1 frankfurter	45	617
Duck, roasted, flesh and skin	½ duck	382	227
Goose, roasted, flesh and skin	½ goose	774	543
Rabbit:			
Leg, raw	4 oz	113	40
Flesh, cooked	4 oz	113	70
Turkey, small, roasted:			
Breast with skin	½ breast	344	182
Leg with skin	1 leg	245	195
Sausages, luncheon meats, and spreads:			
Beer salami, beef	1 slice	6	56
Bologna:			
Beef	1 slice	22	220
Beef and pork	1 slice	22	224
Bratwurst, cooked	1 oz	28	158
Braunschweiger	1 slice	28	324
Brotwurst	1 oz	28	315
Chicken spread	1 oz	28	115
Frankfurter	1 frankfurter	57	639
Ham:			
And cheese loaf	1 oz	28	381
Chopped	1 slice	21	288
Deviled	1 oz	28	253
Spread	1 oz	28	258
Kielbasa	1 slice	26	280
Knockwurst	1 link	68	687
Lebanon bologna	1 slice	18	228
Liver cheese	1 slice	20	245
Old fashioned loaf	1 slice	22	275
Olive loaf	1 slice	21	312
Pepperoni	1 slice	6	122

Food	Portion	Weight (grams)	Sodium (milligrams)
Salami:			
Cooked:			
Beef	1 slice	22	255
Beef and pork	1 slice	22	234
Dry or hard, pork	1 slice	10	226
Sausage:			
Cooked:			
Pork	1 link	13	168
Pork and beef	1 patty	27	217
Smoked	1 link	28	264
Thuringer	1 slice	22	320
Tuna spread	1 oz	28	92
Turkey roll	1 oz	28	166
Vienna sausage	1 link	16	152
Prepared main dishes:			
Beef:			
And macaroni:			
Frozen	6 oz	170	673
Canned	1 cup	227	1,185
Cabbage, stuffed, frozen	8 oz	226	63
Chili con carne with beans, canned:			
Regular	1 cup	255	1,194
Low sodium	1 cup	335	100
Dinners, frozen:			
Beef	1 dinner	312	998
Meat loaf	1 dinner	312	1,304
Sirloin, chopped	1 dinner	284	978
Swiss steak	1 dinner	284	682
Enchiladas	1 pkg	207	725
Goulash, canned	8 oz	227	1,032
Hash, corned beef, canned	1 cup	220	1,520
Meatballs, Swedish	8 oz	227	1,880
Peppers, stuffed, frozen	8 oz	226	1,001
Pizza, frozen:			
With pepperoni	½ pie	195	813
With sausage	½ pie	189	967

Food	Portion	Weight (grams)	Sodium (milli-grams)
Potpie:			
Home baked	1 pie	227	644
Frozen	1 pie	227	1,093
Ravioli, canned	7.5 oz	213	1,065
Spaghetti, canned:			
And ground beef	7.5 oz	213	1,054
And meatballs	7.5 oz	213	942
Sauce	4 oz	114	856
Stew, canned	8 oz	227	980
Chicken:			
And dumplings, frozen	12 oz	340	1,506
And noodles, frozen	¾ cup	180	662
Chow mein, home recipe	1 cup	250	718
Dinner, frozen	1 dinner	312	1,153
Pot pie:			
Home recipe	1 pie	232	594
Frozen	1 pie	227	907
Fish and shellfish:			
Fish dinner, frozen	1 dinner	248	1,212
Shrimp:			
Dinner, frozen	1 dinner	223	758
Egg roll, frozen	1 roll	71	648
Tuna, pot pie, frozen	1 pie	227	715
Pork, sweet and sour canned	1 cup	275	1,968
Turkey:			
Dinner, frozen	1 dinner	333	1,228
Pot Pie:			
Home recipe	1 pie	227	620
Frozen	1 pie	233	1,018
Veal Parmigiana	7.5 oz	214	1,825
Without meat:			
Chow mein, vegetable, frozen	1 cup	240	1,273
Pizza, cheese	¼ 12-in pie	90	447
Spanish rice, canned	1 cup	221	1,370
Fast foods:			
Cheeseburger	1 each	111	709
Chicken dinner	1 portion	410	2,243

Food	Portion	Weight (grams)	Sodium (milligrams)
Fish sandwich	1 sandwich	164	882
French fries	2½ oz	69	146
Hamburger:			
Regular	1 each	92	461
Jumbo	1 each	236	990
Frankfurter	1 frankfurter	93	728
Pizza, cheese	¼ pie	110	599
Shake	1 shake	308	266
Taco	1 taco	75	401

Fruits

Food	Portion	Weight (grams)	Sodium (milligrams)
Apples:			
Raw or baked	1 apple	138	2
Frozen, slices	1 cup	200	28
Frozen, scalloped	8 oz	227	45
Dried, sulfured	8 oz	227	210
Applesauce, canned:			
Sweetened	1 cup	250	6
Unsweetened	1 cup	250	5
With added salt	1 cup	250	68
Apricots:			
Raw	3 apricots	114	1
Canned:			
Peeled	1 cup	258	27
Unpeeled	1 cup	258	10
Dried	1 cup	130	12
Avocado, raw	1 avocado	216	22
Banana, raw	1 banana	119	2
Berries:			
Blackberries (Boysenberries)			
Raw	1 cup	144	1
Canned	1 cup	244	3
Blueberries:			
Raw	1 cup	145	1
Canned	1 cup	250	2

Food	Portion	Weight (grams)	Sodium (milligrams)
Raspberries:			
Raw	1 cup	123	1
Frozen	1 package	284	3
Strawberries:			
Raw	1 cup	149	2
Frozen, sliced	1 cup	255	6
Cherries:			
Raw	1 cup	150	1
Frozen	8 oz	227	3
Canned	1 cup	257	10
Citrus:			
Grapefruit:			
Raw	½ grapefruit	120	1
Frozen, unsweetened	1 cup	244	6
Canned, sweetened	1 cup	254	4
Kumquat	1 kumquat	19	1
Lemon, raw	1 lemon	74	1
Oranges, raw	1 orange	131	1
Tangelo	1 tangelo	95	1
Tangerine	1 tangerine	86	1
Cranberry, raw	1 cup	95	1
Cranberry sauce	1 cup	277	75
Currant:			
Raw	1 cup	133	3
Dried	1 cup	140	10
Dates, dried	10 dates	80	1
Figs:			
Raw	1 fig	50	2
Canned	1 cup	248	3
Dried	1 fig	20	2
Fruit cocktail, canned	1 cup	255	15
Grapes, Thompson seedless	10 grapes	50	1
Mangos, raw	1 mango	200	1
Muskmelon:			
Cantaloup	½ melon	272	24
Casaba	⅛ melon	230	34
Honeydew	⅛ melon	298	28

Food	Portion	Weight (grams)	Sodium (milligrams)
Nectarines, raw	1 nectarine	138	1
Papaya, raw	1 papaya	303	8
Peaches:			
Raw	1 peach	100	1
Frozen	1 cup	250	10
Canned	1 cup	256	15
Dried, uncooked	1 cup	160	10
Pears:			
Raw	1 pear	168	1
Canned	1 cup	255	15
Dried	1 cup	180	10
Pineapple:			
Raw	1 cup	135	1
Canned	1 cup	255	7
Plums:			
Raw	1 plum	66	1
Canned	1 cup	256	10
Prunes:			
Cooked	1 cup	213	8
Dried	5 large	43	2
Raisins, seedless	1 cup	145	17
Rhubarb:			
Cooked, sugared	1 cup	270	5
Frozen	1 cup	270	5
Watermelon	1/16 melon	426	8

Grain Products

Food	Portion	Weight (grams)	Sodium (milligrams)
Barley, pearled, cooked	1 cup	200	6
Biscuits, baking powder:			
Regular flour	1 biscuit	28	175
Self rising flour	1 biscuit	28	185
With milk from mix	1 biscuit	28	272
Low sodium	1 biscuit	28	1
Bread:			
Boston brown	1 slice	45	120
Corn, homemade	1 oz	28	176
Cracked wheat	1 slice	25	148

Food	Portion	Weight (grams)	Sodium (milligrams)
French	1 slice	23	116
Mixed grain	1 slice	23	138
Pita	1 loaf	64	132
Rye:			
Regular	1 slice	25	139
Pumpernickel	1 slice	32	182
Salt rising	1 slice	26	66
White:			
Regular	1 slice	25	114
Thin	1 slice	16	79
Low sodium	1 slice	23	7
Whole wheat	1 slice	25	132
Breakfast cereals:			
Hot, cooked, in unsalted water:			
Corn (hominy) grits:			
Regular	1 cup	236	1
Instant	¾ cup	177	354
Cream of Wheat:			
Regular	¾ cup	184	2
Instant	¾ cup	184	5
Quick	¾ cup	184	126
Mix 'n eat	¾ cup	184	350
Farina	¾ cup	184	1
Oatmeal:			
Regular or quick	¾ cup	180	1
Instant:			
No sodium added	¾ cup	180	1
Sodium added	¾ cup	180	283
With apples and cinnamon	¾ cup	180	220
With maple and brown sugar	¾ cup	180	277
With raisins and spice	¾ cup	180	223
Ready-to eat:			
Bran cereals:			
All-Bran	⅓ cup	28	160
Bran Chex	⅔ cup	28	262
40% Bran	⅔ cup	28	251

Food	Portion	Weight (grams)	Sodium (milli-grams)
100% Bran	½ cup	28	221
Raisin Bran	½ cup	28	209
Cheerios	1 ¼ cup	28	304
Corn cereals:			
Corn Chex	1 cup	28	297
Corn flakes:			
Low sodium	1 ¼ cup	28	10
Regular	1 cup	28	256
Sugar coated	¾ cup	28	274
Sugar Corn Pops	1 cup	28	105
Granola:			
Regular	¼ cup	34	61
No sodium added	¼ cup	34	16
Kix	1½ cup	28	261
Life	⅔ cup	28	146
Product 19	¾ cup	28	175
Rice cereals:			
Low sodium	1 cup	28	10
Puffed rice	2 cups	28	2
Rice Chex	1 ⅛ cup	28	238
Rice Krispies	1 cup	28	340
Sugar coated	⅞ cup	28	149
Special K	1¼ cup	28	265
Total	1 cup	28	359
Trix	1 cup	28	160
Wheat cereals:			
Puffed wheat	2 cups	28	2
Sugar coated	1 cup	28	46
Shredded wheat	1 biscuit	24	3
Wheat Chex	⅔ cup	28	190
Wheaties	1 cup	28	355
Wheat germ, toasted	¼ cup	28	1
Breakfast sweets:			
Coffee cake:			
Almond	⅛ cake	42	167
Blueberry	⅛ cake	35	135
Honey nut	⅛ cake	55	110
Pecan	⅛ cake	40	172

Food	Portion	Weight (grams)	Sodium (milligrams)
Danish:			
Apple, frozen	1 roll	72	220
Cheese, frozen	1 roll	72	250
Cinnamon, frozen	1 roll	72	260
Orange, refrigerated dough	1 roll	39	329
Doughnut:			
Cake type	1 doughnut	32	160
Yeast leavened	1 doughnut	42	99
Sweet rolls:			
Apple crunch, frozen	1 roll	28	105
Caramel, frozen	1 roll	29	118
Cinnamon, frozen	1 roll	26	110
Honey	1 roll	28	119
Toaster pastry:			
Apple, frosted	1 pastry	52	324
Blueberry, frosted	1 pastry	52	242
Cinnamon, frosted	1 pastry	52	326
Strawberry	1 pastry	52	238
Cakes, from mix:			
Angel food:			
Regular	1/12 cake	56	134
One step	1/12 cake	57	250
Devils food	1/12 cake	67	402
Pound	1/12 cake	55	171
White	1/12 cake	68	238
Yellow	1/12 cake	69	242
Cookies:			
Brownies, iced	1 brownie	32	69
Chocolate chip	2 cookies	21	69
Fig bars	2 bars	28	96
Ginger snaps	4 cookies	28	161
Macaroons	2 cookies	38	14
Oatmeal:			
Plain	1 cookie	18	77
With chocolate chips	2 cookies	26	54
With raisins	2 cookies	26	55
Sandwich type	2 cookies	20	96
Shortbread	4 cookies	30	116
Sugar	1 cookie	26	108

Food	Portion	Weight (grams)	Sodium (milligrams)
Sugar wafer	4 cookies	28	43
Vanilla wafer	6 cookies	24	53
Crackers:			
Graham	1 cracker	7	48
Low sodium	1 cracker	4	1
Rye	1 cracker	6	70
Saltine	2 crackers	6	70
Whole wheat	1 cracker	4	30
Macaroni, cooked	1 cup	140	2
Muffin, English	1 medium	57	293
Noodles, cooked	1 cup	140	2
Pancakes, from mix	1 pancake	27	152
Pancake mix	1 cup	141	2,036
Pies, frozen:			
Apple	⅛ of pie	71	208
Banana cream	⅙ of pie	66	90
Bavarian cream:			
Chocolate	⅛ of pie	80	78
Lemon	⅛ of pie	83	71
Blueberry	⅛ of pie	71	163
Cherry	⅛ of pie	71	169
Chocolate cream	⅙ of pie	66	107
Coconut:			
Cream	⅙ of pie	66	104
Custard	⅛ of pie	71	194
Lemon cream	⅙ of pie	66	92
Mince	⅛ of pie	71	258
Peach	⅛ of pie	71	169
Pecan	⅛ of pie	71	241
Pumpkin	⅛ of pie	71	169
Strawberry cream	⅙ of pie	66	101
Rice, cooked:			
Brown	1 cup	195	10
White:			
Regular	1 cup	205	6
Parboiled	1 cup	175	4
Quick	1 cup	165	13
Rolls:			
Brown and serve	1 roll	28	138

Food	Portion	Weight (grams)	Sodium (milligrams)
Refrigerated dough	1 roll	35	342
Snacks:			
Corn chips	1 oz	28	231
Popcorn:			
Caramel coated	1 cup	35	262
Oil, salt	1 cup	9	175
Plain	1 cup	6	1
Potato chips	10 chips	20	200
Pretzels:			
Regular twist	1 pretzel	6	101
Small stick	3 sticks	1	17
Spaghetti, cooked	1 cup	140	2
Stuffing mix, cooked	1 cup	170	1,131
Waffle, frozen	1 waffle	37	275

Legumes and Nuts

Food	Portion	Weight (grams)	Sodium (milligrams)
Almonds:			
Salted, roasted	1 cup	157	311
Unsalted, slivered	1 cup	115	4
Beans:			
Baked, canned:			
Boston style	1 cup	260	606
With or without pork	1 cup	260	928
Dry, cooked:			
Great Northern	1 cup	179	5
Lima	1 cup	192	4
Kidney	1 cup	182	4
Navy	1 cup	195	3
Pinto	1 cup	207	4
Kidney, canned	1 cup	255	844
Brazil nuts, shelled	1 cup	140	1
Cashews:			
Roasted in oil	1 cup	140	21
Dry roasted, salted	1 cup	140	1,200
Chestnuts	1 cup	160	10
Chickpeas, cooked	1 cup	169	13

Food	Portion	Weight (grams)	Sodium (milligrams)
Filberts (hazelnuts) chopped	1 cup	115	2
Lentils, cooked	1 cup	188	4
Peanuts:			
Dry roasted, salted	1 cup	144	986
Roasted, salted	1 cup	144	601
Spanish, salted	1 cup	144	823
Unsalted	1 cup	144	8
Peanut butter:			
Smooth or crunchy	1 tbsp	16	81
Low sodium	1 tbsp	16	1
Peas:			
Blackeye, cooked	1 cup	204	12
Split, cooked	1 cup	237	5
Pecans	1 cup	118	1
Pilinuts	4 oz	113	3
Pistachios	1 cup	125	6

Sugars and Sweets

Food	Portion	Weight (grams)	Sodium (milligrams)
Candy:			
Candy corn	1 oz	28	60
Caramel	1 oz	28	74
Chocolate:			
Bitter	1 oz	28	4
Milk	1 oz	28	28
Fudge, chocolate	1 oz	28	54
Gum drops	1 oz	28	10
Hard	1 oz	28	9
Jelly beans	1 oz	28	3
Licorice	1 oz	28	28
Marshmallows	1 oz	28	11
Mints, uncoated	1 oz	28	56
Peanut brittle	1 oz	28	145
Taffy	1 oz	28	88
Toffee bar, almond	1 oz	28	65
Jams and jellies:			
Jam:			
Regular	1 tbsp	20	2
Low calorie	1 tbsp	20	19

Food	Portion	Weight (grams)	Sodium (milligrams)
Jelly:			
Regular	1 tbsp	18	3
Low calorie	1 tbsp	18	21
Syrup:			
Chocolate flavored:			
Thin	1 tbsp	19	10
Fudge	1 tbsp	19	17
Corn	1 tbsp	20	14
Maple:			
Regular	1 tbsp	20	1
Imitation	1 tbsp	20	20
Molasses:			
Light	1 tbsp	20	3
Medium	1 tbsp	20	7
Blackstrap	1 tbsp	20	18
Sugar:			
Brown	1 cup	220	66
Granulated	1 cup	200	2
Powdered	1 cup	120	1

Vegetables, Vegetable Juices and Salads

Food	Portion	Weight (grams)	Sodium (milligrams)
Artichokes:			
Cooked	1 medium	120	36
Hearts, frozen	3 oz	85	40
Asparagus:			
Raw	1 spear	20	1
Frozen	4 spears	60	4
Canned:			
Regular	4 spears	80	298
Low sodium	1 cup	235	7
Beans:			
Italian:			
Frozen	3 oz	85	4
Canned	1 cup	220	913

Food	Portion	Weight (grams)	Sodium (milli-grams)
Lima:			
Cooked ----------------------	1 cup ---------	170	2
Frozen -----------------------	1 cup ---------	170	128
Canned -----------------------	1 cup ---------	170	456
Low sodium -------------	1 cup ---------	170	7
Snap:			
Cooked -----------------------	1 cup ---------	125	5
Frozen:			
Regular ------------------	3 oz ------------	85	3
With almonds ----------	3 oz ------------	85	335
With mushrooms ------	3 oz ------------	85	145
With onions -------------	3 oz ------------	85	360
Canned:			
Regular ------------------	1 cup ---------	130	326
Low sodium -------------	1 cup ---------	135	3
Beansprouts, mung:			
Raw ------------------------------	1 cup ---------	105	5
Canned --------------------------	1 cup ---------	125	71
Beets:			
Cooked ---------------------------	1 cup ---------	170	73
Canned:			
Sliced ------------------------	1 cup ---------	170	479
Low sodium -----------------	1 cup ---------	170	110
Harvard ----------------------	1 cup ---------	170	275
Pickled -----------------------	1 cup ---------	170	330
Beet greens, cooked ---------------	1 cup ---------	145	110
Broccoli:			
Raw -------------------------------	1 stalk --------	151	23
Frozen:			
Cooked -----------------------	1 cup ---------	188	35
With cheese cause ---------	3.3 oz ---------	94	440
With hollandaise sauce ---	3.3 oz ---------	94	115
Brussels sprouts:			
Raw -------------------------------	1 medium ----	18	1
Frozen:			
Cooked -----------------------	1 cup ---------	150	15
In butter sauce -------------	3.3 oz ---------	94	421

Food	Portion	Weight (grams)	Sodium (milligrams)
Cabbage:			
Green:			
Raw	1 cup	70	8
Cooked	1 cup	144	16
Red, raw	1 cup	70	18
Carrots:			
Raw	1 carrot	72	34
Frozen:			
Cut or whole	3.3 oz	94	43
In butter sauce	3.3oz	94	350
With brown sugar glaze	3.3 oz	94	500
Canned:			
Regular	1 cup	155	386
Low sodium	1 cup	150	58
Cauliflower:			
Raw	1 cup	115	17
Cooked	1 cup	125	13
Frozen:			
Cooked	1 cup	180	18
With cheese sauce	3 oz	85	325
Celery, raw	1 stalk	20	25
Chard, cooked	1 cup	166	143
Chicory	1 cup	90	6
Collards:			
Cooked	1 cup	190	24
Frozen	3 oz	85	41
Corn:			
Cooked	1 ear	140	1
Frozen	1 cup	166	7
Canned:			
Cream style			
Regular	1 cup	256	671
Low sodium	1 cup	256	5
Vacuum pack	1 cup	210	577
Whole kernel:			
Regular	1 cup	165	384
Low sodium	1 cup	166	2
Cucumber	7 slices	28	2
Dandelion greens, cooked	1 cup	105	46

Food	Portion	Weight (grams)	Sodium (milligrams)
Eggplant, cooked	1 cup	200	2
Endive, raw	1 cup	50	7
Kale:			
Cooked	1 cup	110	47
Frozen	3 oz	85	13
Kohlrabi, cooked	1 cup	165	9
Leek	1 bulb	25	1
Lettuce	1 cup	55	4
Mushrooms:			
Raw	1 cup	70	7
Canned	2 oz	56	242
Mustard greens:			
Raw	1 cup	33	11
Cooked	1 cup	140	25
Frozen	3 oz	85	25
Okra, cooked	10 pods	106	2
Onions:			
Mature, dry	1 medium	100	10
Green	2 medium	30	2
Flaked	1 tbsp	6	31
Parsley, raw	1 tbsp	4	2
Parsnips, cooked	1 cup	155	19
Peas, green:			
Cooked	1 cup	160	2
Frozen:			
Regular	3 oz	85	80
In butter sauce	3.3 oz	94	402
In cream sauce	2.6 oz	74	420
With mushrooms	3.3 oz	94	240
Canned:			
Regular	1 cup	170	493
Low sodium	1 cup	170	8
Peppers:			
Hot, raw	1 pod	28	7
Sweet, raw or cooked	1 pod	74	9
Potatoes:			
Baked or boiled	1 medium	156	5

Food	Portion	Weight (grams)	Sodium (milli-grams)
Frozen:			
French fried	10 strips	50	15
Salted	2.5 oz	71	270
Canned	1 cup	250	753
Instant, reconstituted	1 cup	210	485
Mashed, milk and salt	1 cup	210	632
Au gratin	1 cup	245	1,095
Pumpkin, canned	1 cup	245	12
Radish	4 small	18	2
Rutabaga, cooked	1 cup	200	8
Sauerkraut, canned	1 cup	235	1,554
Shallot	1 shallot	20	3
Spinach:			
Raw	1 cup	55	49
Cooked	1 cup	180	94
Frozen:			
Regular	3.3 oz	94	65
Creamed	3 oz	85	280
Canned:			
Regular	1 cup	205	910
Low sodium	1 cup	205	148
Squash:			
Summer:			
Cooked	1 cup	210	5
Frozen, with curry	⅓ cup	71	228
Canned	1 cup	210	785
Winter:			
Baked, mashed	1 cup	205	2
Frozen	1 cup	200	4
Sweetpotatoes:			
Baked or boiled in skin	1 potato	132	20
Canned:			
Regular	1 potato	100	48
Low sodium	1 serving	113	27
Candied	1 potato	100	42
Yam, white, raw	1 cup	200	28
Tomatoes:			
Raw	1 tomato	123	14
Cooked	1 cup	240	10

Food	Portion	Weight (grams)	Sodium (milligrams)
Canned:			
Whole	1 cup	240	390
Stewed	1 cup	240	584
Low sodium	1 cup	240	16
Tomato juice:			
Regular	1 cup	243	878
Low sodium	1 cup	243	9
Tomato paste	1 cup	258	77
Tomato sauce	1 cup	248	1,498
Turnip greens, cooked	1 cup	155	17
Vegetables, mixed:			
Frozen	3.3 oz	94	45
Canned	1 cup	170	380
Vegetable juice cocktail	1 cup	243	887
Salads:			
Bean:			
Marinated	½ cup	130	104
Canned	½ cup	130	537
Carrot-raisin	½ cup	63	97
Cole slaw	½ cup	60	68
Macaroni	⅔ cup	127	676
Potato	½ cup	125	625

Condiments, Fats and Oils

Food	Portion	Weight (grams)	Sodium (milligrams)
Baking powder	1 tsp	3	339
Baking soda	1 tsp	3	821
Catsup:			
Regular	1 tbsp	15	156
Low sodium	1 tbsp	15	3
Chili powder	1 tsp	3	26
Garlic:			
Powder	1 tsp	3	1
Salt	1 tsp	6	1,850
Horse radish, prepared	1 tbsp	18	198
Meat tenderizer:			
Regular	1 tsp	5	1,750
Low sodium	1 tsp	5	1

Food	Portion	Weight (grams)	Sodium (milligrams)
MSG (monosodium glutamate)	1 tsp	5	492
Mustard, prepared	1 tsp	5	65
Olives:			
Green	4 olives	16	323
Ripe, mission	3 olives	15	96
Onion:			
Powder	1 tsp	2	1
Salt	1 tsp	5	1,620
Parsley, dried	1 tbsp	1	6
Pepper, black	1 tsp	2	1
Pickles:			
Bread and butter	2 slices	15	101
Dill	1 pickle	65	928
Sweet	1 pickle	15	128
Relish, sweet	1 tbsp	15	124
Salt	1 tsp	5	1,938
Sauces:			
A-1	1 tbsp	17	275
Barbecue	1 tbsp	16	130
Chili:			
Regular	1 tbsp	17	227
Low sodium	1 tbsp	15	11
Soy	1 tbsp	18	1,029
Tabasco	1 tsp	5	24
Tartar	1 tbsp	14	182
Teriyaki	1 tbsp	18	690
Worcestershire	1 tbsp	17	206
Vinegar	½ cup	120	1
Yeast, baker's, dry	1 package	7	1
Fats, oils, and related products:			
Butter:			
Regular	1 tbsp	14	116
Unsalted	1 tbsp	14	2
Whipped	1 tbsp	9	74
Margarine:			
Regular	1 tbsp	14	140
Unsalted	1 tbsp	14	1
Oil, vegetable, (includes corn,		14	0
olive, and soybean)	1 tbsp	14	0

Food	Portion	Weight (grams)	Sodium (milli-grams)
Salad dressing:			
Blue cheese	1 tbsp	15	153
French:			
Home recipe	1 tbsp	14	92
Bottled	1 tbsp	14	214
Dry mix, prepared	1 tbsp	14	253
Low sodium	1 tbsp	15	3
Italian:			
Bottled	1 tbsp	15	116
Dry mix, prepared	1 tbsp	14	172
Mayonnaise	1 tbsp	15	78
Russian	1 tbsp	15	133
Thousand Island:			
Regular	1 tbsp	16	109
Low cal	1 tbsp	14	153

Index

196

Meat, 93
Meat, salt in, 28
Medical College of Wisconsin, 99
Menopause, 17, 18
Mességué, Maurice, 81
Miami, University of, 138
Michigan, University of, 109, 127
Milk, 27, 30
Minerals (see also individual
    minerals), 40ff., 117
Mississippi, University of,
    Medical School, 34
Mitschek, Dr. G. H., 84
Morales, Betty Lee, 142

N

National Cancer Institute, 156
National Enquirer, 22
The National Hog Farmer, 52
National Research Council, 52
Nebraska, University of, 153, 156
*New England Journal of
    Medicine*, 98
New York Times, 15, 19
Niacin (see "Vitamin B3")
Nieper, Dr. Hans, 45
Nitrates, 95
Noise, 138
Northwestern University, 10
Nutrition (see also "Diet"), 22
Nutrition Against Disease, 69, 86
Nutrition Reviews, 80
Nutrition Today, 125
*Nutritional Factors in General
    Medicine*, 110

O

Ochsner, Dr. Alton, 63, 65
Onions, 79
Overweight, 21
Oxford University, England, 21
Oxygen, 69

P

Pancreas, 87
Pantothenic acid, 151
Parsley, 79
Pauling, Dr. Linus, 63, 70
Pectin, 84, 85
Physiology Review, 118
Posner, Dr. Howard, 82
Potassium, 20, 34ff., 45, 46, 47,
    79, 117, 118, 146
Potassium, amount in foods, 164
Preservatives, 31, 87, 95
Prevention, 35, 82, 96
Preventive Medicine, 93
Processing of foods, 60
Prostate gland, 53, 98
Protein, 125
Prutting, Dr. John, 47
The Pulse Test, 97

R

Reserpine, 21
Ringsdorf, Dr. W. M., Jr., 41
Roosevelt, Eleanor, 77
Rosenman, Dr. Ray H., 116
Russek, Dr. Henry I., 138
Rutgers University, 85

S

St. Vincent's Hospital, Montclair,
    N.J., 42
Saccharin, 91
Sacrum, 161

Weight (see also "Overweight"), 122
Western Reserve University, 152
Wheat, 96
Wheat germ, 54
Whey, 83
Williams, Dr. Roger, 69, 71, 86, 105, 108, 128, 151, 157
Wood, Dr. Randall, 154
Women, 17, 40
World Health Organization, 147

YZ

Yoga, 141
Yogurt, 84, 85
Yudkin, Dr. John, 89, 129
Zinc, 51ff., 88, 111, 147
Zinc, amount needed daily, 55
Zinc, food sources of, 54
Zofehak, Dr. George, 81

Read What the Experts Say About Larchmont Books!

Megavitamin Therapy

"This book provides a much-needed perspective about the relationship of an important group of medical and psychiatric conditions, all of which seem to have a common causation (the grossly improper American Diet) and the nutritional techniques which have proven to be of great benefit in their management."—*Robert Atkins, M.D., author of "Dr. Atkins' Diet Revolution," New York.*

"This responsible book gathers together an enormous amount of clinical and scientific data and presents it in a clear and documented way which is understandable to the average reader... The authors have provided critical information plus references for the acquisition of even more essential knowledge."—*David R. Hawkins, M.D., The North Nassau Mental Health Center, Manhasset, New York.*

Health Foods

"This book (and "Is Low Blood Sugar Making You a Nutritional Cripple") are companion books worth adding to your library. The fact that one of the books is labeled "health foods" is an indication how far our national diet has drifted away from those ordinary foods to which man has adapted over the past million years...."—*A. Hoffer, M.D., Ph.D., The Huxley Newsletter.*

"A sensible, most enlightening review of foods and their special qualities for maintenance of health...."—*The Homeostasis Quarterly.*

*The best books on health
and nutrition are from*

LARCHMONT BOOKS

Vitamin B12 and Folic Acid, by Adams and Murray, 176 pages, $1.95.

Vitamin C, The Powerhouse Vitamin, Conquers More than Just Colds, by Adams and Murray, Foreword by Dr. Frederick R. Klenner, 192 pages, $1.50.

Vitamin E, Wonder Worker of the 70's?, by Adams and Murray, Foreword by Dr. Evan V. Shute, 192 pages, $1.25.

Titles from

THE PREVENTIVE HEALTH LIBRARY

Improving Your Health with Vitamin A, by Adams and Murray, 128 pages, $1.25.

Improving Your Health with Vitamin C, by Adams and Murray, 160 pages, $1.50.

Improving Your Health with Vitamin E, by Adams and Murray, 176 pages, $1.50.

Improving Your Health with Calcium and Phosphorous, by Adams and Murray, 128 pages, $1.25.

Improving Your Health with Niacin (Vitamin B$_3$), by Adams and Murray, 128 pages, $1.25.

Improving Your Health with Zinc, by Adams and Murray, 128 pages, $1.50.